personal
fitness

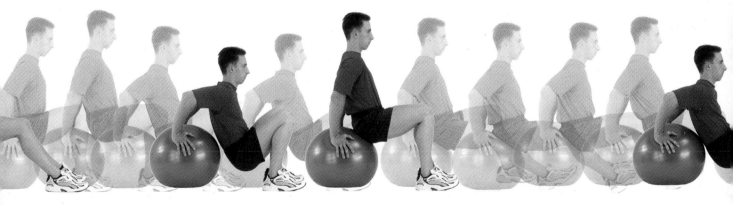

a *flow*motion™ title

personal
fitness

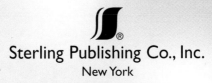

simon frost

Sterling Publishing Co., Inc.

New York

Created and conceived by
Axis Publishing Limited
8c Accommodation Road
London NW11 8ED
www.axispublishing.co.uk

Creative Director: Siân Keogh
Managing Editor: Matthew Harvey
Project Designer: Anna Knight
Project Editor: Louise Aikman, Michael Spilling
Production Manager: Sue Bayliss
Photographer: Mike Good

Library of Congress Cataloging-in-Publication
Data Available

10 9 8 7 6 5 4 3 2 1

Published in 2002 by Sterling Publishing Co., Inc.
387 Park Avenue South, New York, NY 10016
Text and images © Axis Publishing Limited 2002
Distributed in Canada by Sterling Publishing
C/o Canadian Manda Group,
One Atlantic Avenue, Suite 105
Toronto, Ontario, M6K 3E7, Canada

Separation by United Graphics Pte Limited
Printed and bound by Star Standard (Pte) Limited

Sterling ISBN 0–8069–8879–7

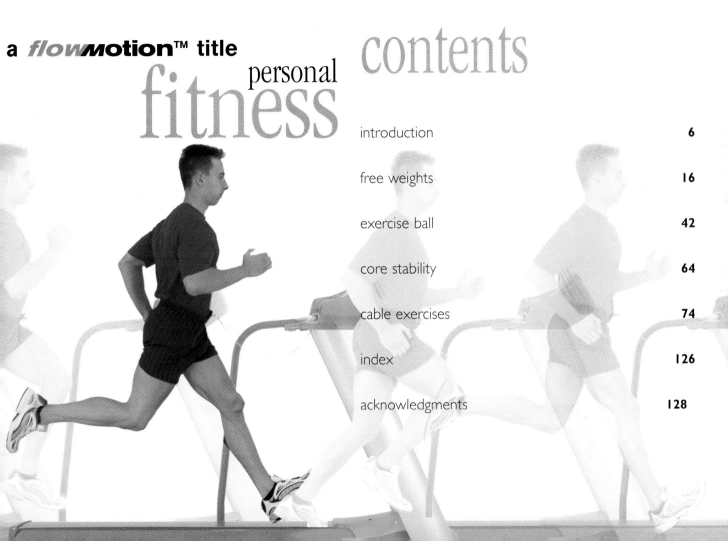

a *flowmotion*™ title

fitness personal

contents

basics of resistance training

The term resistance training (also known as strength training or weight training) is a simple description of a type of exercise that uses the body's muscular system to move against an opposing force. This force can be created in various ways using machines, free weights, exercise balls, dynabands, natural body weight, and even running. This book covers a whole range of equipment and provides detailed descriptions of correct technique, which is the most important factor to consider when performing such activities. By following the images and using the text as a guide, you will be able to develop the proper technique for resistance training. This foundation will help you to build muscle strength safely.

Every day, more and more people are doing resistance training, but sadly few actually examine the content and structure of their workout. With a well-designed program you can train to achieve much more than just bigger muscles. The benefits of resistance training include not only increased muscle strength, endurance, size, and mass, but also reduced body fat, improved muscle tone, increased metabolism, increased bone density and enhanced sports performance.

understanding the language

Before beginning resistance training, it is important to become familiar with training terms and concepts, as well as some of the main development and safety issues facing exercisers.

ISOMETRIC This refers to a muscle contraction where there is a lack of movement about a joint. This can be achieved by contracting against a resistance (for example, a heavy object), or by contracting against an immovable object (such as a wall or floor). Isometric training is used to increase strength at a particular joint angle. This type of training is useful for overcoming a sticking point, that is, the part of a movement where the muscle is biomechanically at its weakest.

REPETITIONS (reps) These are the number of movements made during a set. A repetition has two phases. The first is called concentric, which refers to a muscle shortening action when a joint angle is decreasing—such as the lifting part of a biceps curl; and eccentric, which refers to the muscle lengthening action when the joint angle is increasing—such as the lowering part of a biceps curl. Repetitions determine training results: Higher reps focus more on endurance and toning, while lower reps have a greater effect on muscle strength and size.

SET This is a group of reps performed continuously. A set can consist of any number of reps, normally up to 20. Sets normally range from 1–10 and, like reps, also affect the training result. More sets produce greater training volume, which will result in greater lean muscle mass, reduced body fat, and increased muscle size. Ideally, the beginner should start with one set of reps, and increase the number of sets once the muscles have been rested; provided they have not reached the point of overload.

STRENGTH This is a muscle's ability to contract maximally against a force. Strength is usually measured by performing one repetition maximally (1RM). Strength can be increased by low-rep, high-intensity weight training and increased volume.

TONE This term describes the appearance of a muscle when rested. The more toned a muscle is, the greater the muscle density and firmness. A toned muscle may appear tight, but it can be equally as supple as an intoned muscle.

ENDURANCE This refers to a muscle's ability to contract continuously until fatigue affects the technique or you cannot perform the movement any more. Repeating movements to overload and increasing volume can improve endurance. There is a connection between strength and endurance, in that you cannot get stronger without some sort of increase in endurance. For example, if someone were to train at three sets of six to eight reps to enhance strength, the maximum endurance of 15 reps would also improve. Although the gain in endurance would not be as dramatic as the strength gain, it would be enough to create an easier high rep performance.

HYPERTROPHY This indicates an increase in the muscle fiber size. Improved hypertrophy is the aim of many bodybuilding programs; it is achieved with low-rep, high-intensity, and volume exercise.

SPECIFICITY In order for a muscle to gain from a training effect, that muscle must be specifically targeted by the exercise. Some exercises involve many muscles, but they still have a focus muscle, where the supporting muscles are assisting the prime mover.

PRIME MOVER During an exercise the main muscle contracting to create the direction of movement is called the prime mover. Some exercises use three different muscles at the same time, there is only one prime mover.

ANTAGONIST This is the term given to the muscle that relaxes while the opposing, contracting muscle creates movement. For example, if the leg is extended the quadriceps are the prime mover and the hamstrings are the antagonistic muscles.

STABILIZER These muscles are responsible for the control factor during an exercise; for example, during a chest press the prime mover is the pectoralis major and the stabilizing muscles are that of the shoulder.

MUSCLE FIBER TYPES Muscles can only pull—they do not push against the bones to which they are attached. Muscles shorten and lengthen with control against resistance, which pulls the weight back to the starting position. Muscles consist of two main muscle fibers.

Slow twitch fibers are small fibers that can produce a low level of force for a longer period of time, and so are used for endurance-based activities. This type of muscle fiber is mostly used during aerobic activity and should be trained by completing high-rep, low-force exercise.

Fast twitch fibers are generally more powerful. These fibers are used for high-force, short duration exercises and are larger than the slow twitch fibers. The fast twitch fibers are exercised by doing high-force, low-rep weight training.

In all weight training exercise both muscle fiber types will always be active regardless of the stimulus, but the predominant fiber will be used according to the demands of the movement. Because the slow twitch fibers are more fatigue-resistant, the body will activate this fiber type first and then move to the fast twitch.

technique

Correct technique is vital if one is to achieve effective results from resistance exercise. It is common for people to aim to lift as heavy a weight as possible. In doing so, they sacrifice good posture to adopt an easier lifting position that allows them to overcome the biomechanical sticking points of certain exercises. This change in posture will affect the prime mover muscle overload and reduce its isolation, thus reducing the potential to achieve specific muscle development. At the same time this will put more emphasis on the stabilizing muscles, transforming the exercise to become a general workout.

SPEED AND RANGE OF MOVEMENT (ROM) Equally important are the speed and range of movement (ROM). Increased speed can promote performance for power training. This usually requires specialized gym equipment that targets specific muscles and muscle groups and is designed to create an even force at a set speed over the entire ROM. Without this style of equipment, speed training has an increased risk of injury. This is due to the excessive forces produced by the speed at which the exercise is performed.

BREATHING This is an essential part of any training technique. Breathing should be done in rhythm with the exercise, exhaling on the initial direction of movement and inhaling on the return. An alternative approach involves inhaling before you start the lift, holding your breath during the lift and then exhaling at the end before inhaling on the return. The first method is the safest and most practical breathing technique, while the second allows you to lift heavier weights as the torso becomes rigid when filled with air. This creates a better lifting platform, but at the risk of increased blood pressure.

Holding the breath is not recommended when doing resistance training, especially while performing exercises that involve overhead movements (such as a shoulder press) and movements where the heart is higher than the head (such as a bench press or French press).

KEEP ON MOVING
Unless you have high blood pressure, try to maintain tension within the active muscles during the movement. Do not allow the active muscles to relax in the starting position, or let the weights rest between reps. While keeping a constant movement avoid locking the joints: A locked joint can become compressed and worn over time.

OVERLOAD This describes an application of force that is greater than a muscle or group of muscles would normally encounter. Overload will produce a physical adaptation, specific to the muscles used to gain the required training effect. Overload must be achieved regardless of the training goal. For example, if fat loss is the goal, the target total calorie expenditure should be greater than the total calories consumed. Overload is the most effective way to achieve results, but must be regular and progressive to avoid unnecessary over training or muscle strain. To achieve overload you do not have to increase the amount of weight lifted; you can increase or decrease the speed, number of sets, reps, and volume.

INTENSITY This is the key to effective overloading. Different kinds of intensity produce different results. For example, if you wish to become more toned in your biceps, you could start a program of three sets of 15 reps and become fatigued by the end of the third set, creating overload. Keen to progress, you might then increase the weight too quickly, causing a reduction in reps down to 10. By increasing the intensity too quickly, the training effect becomes more strength-based.

VOLUME Increasing volume is also a great way to achieve overload. Volume can be increased by adding more reps and sets to a routine, or by adding an extra exercise to the muscle, that is, two biceps exercises per session. Frequent training sessions also increase volume: By working the bicep three times a week rather than two, you can produce greater overload. However there is a relationship between volume and muscle size: The greater the volume, the more likely one's muscles will enter hypertrophy. Volume also plays a very important role in losing fat: Increased volume creates greater muscle mass, which improves the body's metabolic rate. It is recommended that each muscle group should be trained at least twice a week in order to progress.

PERIODIZATION All training must be varied on a regular basis to prevent complete adaptation. If you do not alter or vary your exercise routine, your muscles will cease to overload and no longer develop. Subtle changes in exercise technique, reps, and sets are important to continue to achieve results, whether this be in strength, endurance, or tone.

RECOVERY Between sets there can be temporary muscle fatigue. This is caused by a range of physical factors, like the production of lactic acid, nerve impulse interference, and depleted energy stores. This fatigue is only temporary and will subside with a short rest. The rest between sets and exercises plays an important role in the type of result achieved. If strength is the goal, then longer rests of up to seven minutes should be used. If endurance is the goal, then rest periods might be less than a minute. Generally, recovery between sessions should be one day. There is a lasting form of muscle soreness called delayed onset muscle soreness (DOMS). DOMS usually follows 24–48 hours after the training session and can persist for up to four days. DOMS is a sign of severe overload.

systems

Systems are used to give structure to a workout. They apply the best possible combination of reps, sets, rest, volume, and intensity to achieve the desired outcome. There are many different kinds of systems and a lot of them give similar results. A few are listed here to provide a simple but effective exercise program.

EXERCISE BALL This is an easy way to increase resistance when working a specific muscle group.

SYSTEM	REPS	SETS	FREQUENCY
SINGLE SET STRENGTH, HIGH INTENSITY **BEGINNER**	8–12	1	3 times per week per muscle group
SINGLE SET ENDURANCE, HIGH INTENSITY **BEGINNER**	12–15	1	3 times per week per muscle group
MULTIPLE SET STRENGTH, MEDIUM INTENSITY **INTERMEDIATE–ADVANCED**	5–6	3–7	At least twice per week, depending on recovery
MULTIPLE SET ENDURANCE, MEDIUM INTENSITY **INTERMEDIATE–ADVANCED**	12–15 or 15–20	3–7	At least twice per week, depending on recovery. Rest periods should be 30 secs between sets and exercise.
CIRCUIT, GENERAL INTENSITY **ADVANCED**	10–15	1–3 circuits	2–4 times per week

REST	NOTES
1 min between exercise	Good system for increasing strength and endurance with a minimal increase in size. Ideal for a short workout where the whole body can be trained with 8–10 exercises, taking about 25 mins to complete. Because of the maximal intensity, a good warm-up with a rehearsal set is necessary.
30 secs between exercise	
30 secs between exercise	Generally 3 sets are used, but for advanced body building programs up to 7 can be completed. Normally the weight is constant throughout. With the larger set volume there may be 2 warm-up sets where the weight is increased. Due to the volume the weight is fixed at medium intensity. The strength gains are higher than with single set training, but there is a greater chance of increase in muscle size and the session is longer. The workout can be split into body parts for different days, as the session time might exceed 1½ hours for a whole workout.
30 secs to 1 min **Rest between muscles and exercises. There should be a 1–2 day rest that increases with the number of sets.**	
Rest between exercises should be minimal (15–30 secs). There should be a 1–2 days rest between sessions.	Circuits are a great way to increase strength and endurance. They consist of a series of exercises done in sequence, where each exercise is done to light fatigue. Rest periods are minimal, and the exerciser should not stop until one circuit is complete.

PERIPHERAL HEART ACTION SYSTEM	
SYSTEM	Medium/high intensity, heart rate to be kept above 140 bpm **ADVANCED**
REPS	**Can be done with high or low reps, but normally done between 8-12 reps**
SETS	**3 sets with several sequences**
FREQUENCY	**3 times per week or split into high volume exercise and done 4-5 times per week**
REST	**Minimal between exercises and sequences– 15 secs should be enough.**
NOTES	This is a modified circuit that is more cardiovascular-based. The aim is to keep the heart rate at 140 or above the entire time. In this system the training is split into several routines that contain 4–6 different exercises. The exercises are done in a circuit format, with minimal rest between them. Once up to 3 circuits are completed on all the exercises, the exerciser then moves on to the next sequence until all 7 sequences are complete. This type of training is very tiring, but has great aerobic and muscular endurance benefits.

system rules and safety

splitting

Splitting is a system that can be added to any other system. The reason for splitting is to work harder with higher volume on each muscle group. With splitting, the muscles may require a longer rest period, but they still need to be trained a minimum of once a week. The following are some examples of splitting.

1. Upper body on the first session and lower body on the next. This is good for low volume splits and shorter workouts. This type of split can be done each day as one set of muscles is resting while the others are working.

2. Chest with triceps and shoulders on one day, then biceps, back, and legs on the next. This is good if you want high volume with the aim of improving size or tone. This workout could also be done daily, but with the increased volume, a day's rest after every two workouts may be required.

3. Chest with biceps and legs on the first session, then work with triceps, back, and shoulders on the next. This system will promote better strength gains, as there is no muscle pre-fatigue during the workout. At least one day's rest is required between the two workouts, as the lack of recovery will affect the second workout.

system rules

- Reps should always work in ranges (for example, 8–10), as this allows the muscles to overload within the target zone.

- If you can complete more reps than the target range, then the weight should be increased, and vice versa if the reps are below the range.

- Overload should be achieved, either through fatigue or failure within the target zone.

- The aim should be to stay at a set weight until the higher target is comfortably achieved, that is, 10 out of 8–10 reps. Only then should the weight be increased.

- Sets should be added only after the muscle can perform one set maximally to failure.

- If an extra set is added, it must achieve the target rep range. If it fails to do so, then the muscle is not ready for the extra set.

- Always rest between exercises and sets, otherwise the correct overload will not be achieved.

- Do not exceed 1½ hours of training at a time, as your performance will decline as you become tired.

- With high-volume training, the body should be split into muscle groups (for example, chest and back), but make sure that each muscle is rested for at least a day and the exercises are repeated at least twice a week.

safety

It is vital that you train in a safe environment and use the correct training techniques. Ensure there is plenty of space around you when using free weights. Wear clothing that allows freedom of movement. Also remember to check your posture regularly to avoid possible stress or damage to muscles and ligaments.

OVER TRAINING To get results from weight training one has to achieve the minimum overload for each muscle group. If you train more than three times per week, you could be over training. If the body has not repaired from the previous session, this is because the intensity was too high and the muscle damage continued for too long. If you choose to train intensively, it is best to reduce the frequency to allow more time for the muscles to rest. It is best to train more frequently and less intensively, as this will give a greater training effect. Too much training volume, intensity, or a combination of both can lead to chronic fatigue. The first sign of over training is usually a sudden reduction in performance that will not clear with a few days rest. Over training can be very severe, with both physical and psychological symptoms. Some of the physical signs include decreased body weight, reduced appetite, poor sleep, increased resting heart rate, higher resting blood pressure, muscle soreness, and nausea. Due to individual variations it can be very hard to see the warning signs—it may be that you feel unmotivated, moody, and less confident, or suffer from poor concentration, depression, anger, or irritability.

SPOTTING A spotter is someone who is there to assist the exerciser with a difficult exercise and to summon help if required. When selecting someone to spot you should be sure of the following:

● Good communication between the spotter and exerciser is essential.

● The spotter must be strong enough to lift the weight that the exerciser is using.

● The spotter must be familiar with the exercise technique and the position from which they should spot.

● The spotter should be aware of the exerciser's repetition goal.

● The spotter must be attentive at all times and ready to get help if necessary.

warm up, cool down

GENERAL WARM-UP A warm-up prior to any exercise is necessary to increase body temperature, reduce the chance of muscular stress, prepare the mind, improve coordination, and balance and mobilize the joints. A general warm-up might consist of some kind of low-intensity aerobic training for five to ten minutes and stretching.

PERFORMANCE SPECIFIC WARM-UP We recommend a specific warm-up to prepare for training if high intensity and performance are the objectives. This involves rehearsing the actual exercise but with a decreased intensity and volume. You can also stretch the muscles you intend to exercise as a preparation for resistance training.

COOLING DOWN A cool down should follow any exercise program. To cool down effectively, it is best to do a low-intensity exercise for three to seven minutes. This will help to prevent the effects of blood pooling, where the blood floods the lower extremities and causes a reduced blood flow back to the heart. This can cause faintness, dizziness, and nausea. When the muscles are moving, they help pump blood back to the heart.

HIP FLEXOR STRETCH Place one knee forward and extend your trailing leg behind. Rest your hands on your knee, while keeping your hips square and your upper body vertical.

GROIN STRETCH Holding the soles of your feet together, gently push your knees toward the ground while keeping your back straight.

QUADRICEPS STRETCH *below* Balancing on one leg, pull up the other foot behind your body. Keep your body upright to maximize the stretch through the front of the leg.

ILIOTIBIAL STRETCH *left* Place one foot over the other, with both feet flat on the ground. Keeping both legs straight, lean your hips away from your rear foot. You should feel a stretch down the outside of your leg.

HAMSTRING STRETCH *right* Keep one leg straight. Bend the supporting leg at the knee and rest both hands on your thigh to support your weight. Now bend forwards from the hips, keeping your back straight.

go with the flow

The special *Flowmotion* images used in this book have been created to ensure that you see the whole movement—not just selected highlights. Each of the image sequences flows across the page from left to right, demonstrating how the exercise progresses and how to get into each position safely and effectively. Each exercise is labeled as being suitable for beginners, intermediate, or advanced students by a colored tab above the title. The captions along the bottom of the images provide additional information to help you perform the exercises confidently. Below this, another layer of information is contained in the timeline, including instructions for breathing and symbols indicating when to hold a position.

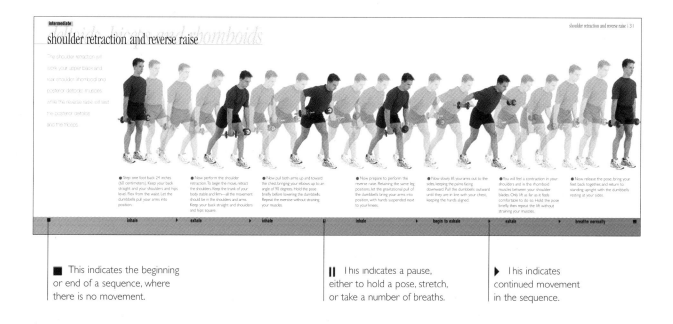

intermediate

shoulder retraction and reverse raise

shoulder retraction and reverse raise | 31

The shoulder retraction will work your upper back and rear shoulder (rhomboid and posterior deltoid) muscles, while the reverse raise will test the posterior deltoids and the triceps.

● Step one foot back 24 inches (60 centimeters). Keep your back straight and your shoulders and hips level. Flex from the waist. Let the dumbbells pull your arms into position.

● Now perform the shoulder retraction. To begin the move, retract the shoulders. Keep the trunk of your body stable and firm—all the movement should be in the shoulders and arms. Keep your back straight and shoulders and hips square.

● Now pull both arms up and toward the chest, bringing your elbows up to an angle of 90 degrees. Hold the pose briefly before lowering the dumbbells. Repeat the exercise without straining your muscles.

● Now prepare to perform the reverse raise. Retaining the same leg positions, let the gravitational pull of the dumbbells bring your arms into position, with hands suspended next to your knees.

● Now slowly lift your arms out to the sides, keeping the palms facing downward. Pull the dumbbells outward until they are in line with your chest, keeping the hands aligned.

● You will feel a contraction in your shoulders and in the rhomboid muscles between your shoulder blades. Only lift as far as it feels comfortable to do so. Hold the pose briefly, then repeat the lift without straining your muscles.

● Now release the pose, bring your feet back together, and return to standing upright with the dumbbells resting at your sides.

■   inhale   ▶   exhale   ▶   inhale   ‖   inhale   ▶   begin to exhale   ▶   exhale   ▶   breathe normally   ■

■ This indicates the beginning or end of a sequence, where there is no movement.

‖ This indicates a pause, either to hold a pose, stretch, or take a number of breaths.

▶ This indicates continued movement in the sequence.

free weights

squats
quadriceps and gluteus maximus

This is a primary exercise for working the quadricep muscles at the front of the thighs. This movement will also test the hamstrings, adductors, and gluteal muscles. The narrow and wider variations will allow you to isolate the quadriceps or adductors.

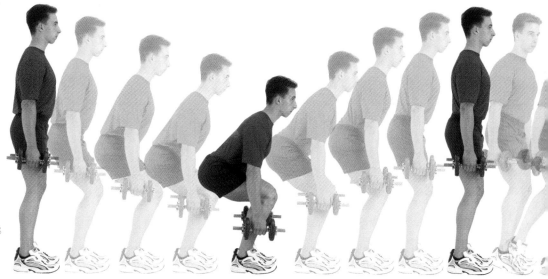

● Stand with your feet shoulder width apart, abdominals tight, and sternum upright. Lower slowly, flexing at the knees. Don't let your knees extend beyond your toes—adjustment should come from your hips to gain the maximum benefit from the movement.

● Lower yourself until your knees are almost 90 degrees. Keep your head up and your back straight, balancing your body on your heels. It is important to keep your pelvis square so that your balance and weight remain central— don't allow the body to tip forward.

● As you lower yourself, the dumbbells should stay slightly forward to maintain balance, but your arms should be relaxed. All the body weight should be on your heels (you should still be able to move your toes).

| exhale | ▶ | begin to inhale | ▶ | inhale | ▶ |

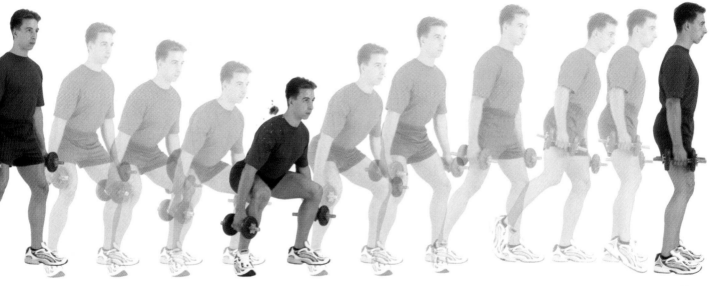

● Moving smoothly, raise yourself slowly back into the start position, raising your bottom and straightening (but not locking) your knees. Now do the squats from a wider leg position, with your feet roughly 24 inches (60 centimeters) apart at the heels.

● Point your toes outward at 45 degrees from the body. Lower yourself again, making sure that your knees track the direction of your feet. Keep your weight centered back on your heels and don't lean forward. Squat until your knees are at 90 degrees.

● Now raise yourself, lifting from the knees. Keep your sternum pointed forward and your back straight throughout the upward movement.

● Return to the starting position, with your arms relaxed at your sides and your legs soft at the knees. Repeat both movements without straining.

exhale   ‖   inhale   ▶   exhale   ▶   breathe normally   ■

dead lifts and lunges *gluteals, and quadriceps*

This sequence consists of two movements that will work the muscles on both the front and back of the thighs. The dead lifts test the hamstring and gluteal muscles while the standing forward lunge works the quadriceps.

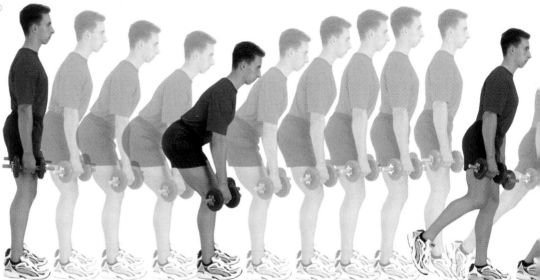

● Hold the weights in a central position throughout the movement and keep your arms at a 45 degree angle to the body. Begin the exercise by flexing at the knees and bending your upper body forward.

● Keep your legs bent and your arms straight, moving the weights to the front of your body as you bend. Take the dumbbells down to just past your knees. Now slowly raise your body. You will feel a contraction in your hamstrings.

● Stand up fully. Keep your back straight and don't arch or hunch your shoulders. All the movement should come from your hips and bottom. Now return to the start position and repeat the dead lift without straining the muscles.

inhale ▶ **begin to exhale** ▶ **exhale**

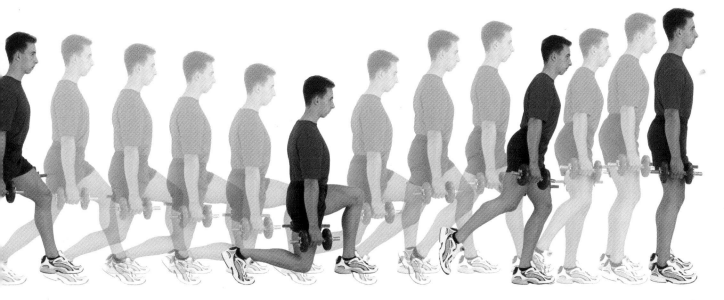

● To set up for the lunge, step your left foot roughly 36 inches (90 centimeters) forward. Keep your back straight and your hips square. Hold the dumbbells loosely at your sides.

● Now inhale and lower yourself, bringing your right knee down toward the floor. Your upper body should stay rigid throughout the movement, so that only the leg muscles are working. Maintain a neutral, upright pelvis.

● Fully extended, your left shin should remain roughly upright and the knee should not extend beyond your toes. The right knee should not touch the floor. Remember not to step forward too far, as this could cause the pelvis to rotate.

● Hold this position for a second, then exhale and step back to the start position. Now repeat the forward lunge on the other leg. Work both legs alternately without straining the muscles.

inhale ▶ inhale ▶ exhale ▶ ■

standing leg extension *and quadriceps*

By pulling against gravity, this simple but effective stretching exercise will work the hamstrings and quardicep muscles. Good balance is essential to perform this exercise effectively, so you may want to stand near a wall for support.

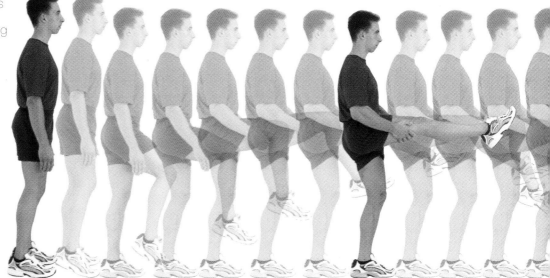

● Slowly raise your right leg, flexing at the hip. Keep your standing leg soft at the knee to remain flexible and balanced throughout the movement. Keep your back straight and your head facing forward.

● Raise your hands to support the back of your right thigh. Now slowly extend the leg from the knee joint. The leg should be approximately 90 degrees to the body. Lean back slightly from the hips to compensate for the weight adjustment.

● Soften your standing leg and extend the right leg as far as you can. You will feel a stretch along the underside of your extended leg and a contraction in the quadriceps. If you can, lock the knee. Keep the sole of the foot flat and do not try to extend the toes.

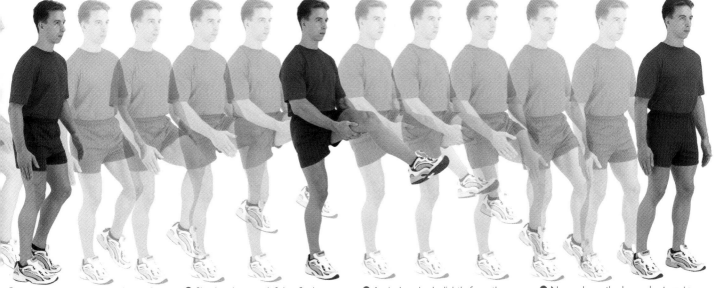

● Now release the contraction and return your leg to the floor. Bring yourself back to the upright standing position. Now repeat the leg extension with the left leg.

● Slowly raise your left leg, flexing at the hip until the leg is 90 degrees to the body. Keep your standing leg soft at the knee to maintain balance. Bring your hands forward and hold the underneath of the left thigh.

● Again, lean back slightly from the hips to compensate for the weight adjustment, tilting your pelvis upward. You will feel a stretch along the underside of your extended leg and a contraction in the quadriceps.

● Now release the leg and return to an upright standing position, with your arms relaxed at your sides and your legs soft at the knees.

inhale ▶ begin to exhale ▶ exhale ▶ breathe normally ∎

seated calf raise

This is a simple but effective way of working your calf muscles. To do this seated variation, you will need a chair to sit on and a step or other raised surface about three inches (eight centimeters) off the ground.

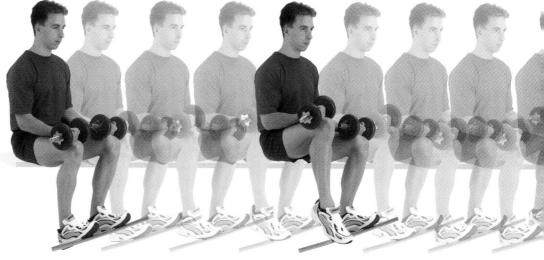

● Sit on the chair with your back upright. Place the balls of your feet on the platform with the heel resting toward the floor. Hold the dumbbells balanced on your knees with your elbows resting on your thighs.

● Perform the exercise on one leg at a time. To begin the movement, push from the ball of your right foot to raise your leg, so that your foot is hinging on the step or platform. Plantarflex your foot to bring the heel up and point the toes downward.

● You will feel a contraction in your calf muscles. Now lower your foot again to the starting position. Do not let the foot drop too low, as this can put a strain on the calf muscles and Achilles tendon.

| inhale | ▶ | begin to exhale | ▶ | exhale |

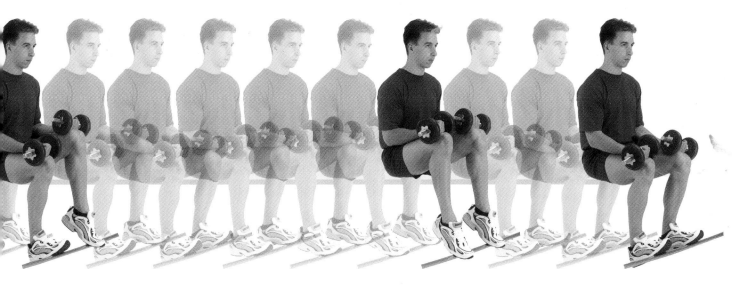

● Now repeat the raise using your left foot. Push from the ball of your left foot to raise your knee. Plantarflex your foot to bring the heel up and point the toes downward. You will feel a contraction in the calf muscles.

● Lower your foot again to the starting position. Now repeat the exercise with both legs simultaneously.

● Push from the balls of both feet to raise the knees. Plantarflex your feet to bring the heels up and point the toes downward. Hold the position briefly, then lower the feet to bring the heels toward the floor.

● You can also do a standing version of the calf raise: balance on the balls of your feet on a step or platform, and using just your body weight, lower and raise yourself, hinging at the ankles.

exhale ▶ **inhale** ❚❚ **exhale** ▶ **breathe normally** ❚❚

chest fly and press
pectoralis and triceps

This series of movements concentrates on the pectoral (chest) muscles, as well as working the shoulders and triceps. It is better to lie flat on the floor rather than using a bench when performing this exercise, as research suggests that lowering your arms beyond the line of the body can damage the muscles.

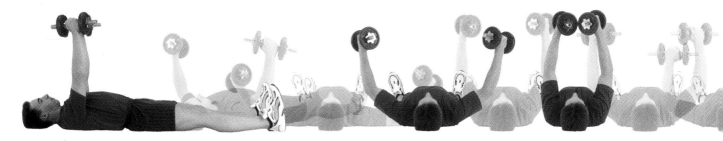

● To set up for the chest fly, lie flat on the floor. Hold the dumbbells firmly with your forearms extended vertically, elbows locked and shoulder flexion at 90 degrees. Your palms should be facing inward toward your body.

● To begin the chest fly, inhale and lower the arms downward, moving the weights in a smooth arc out to your sides. The angles of your elbows should remain constant and even throughout the movement. Bring your elbows down to rest on the floor.

● Now push upward and adduct your arms fully to bring the weights together so that they are touching. Do not lock your arms at the elbows. Hold the pose for a second.

● With the weights held above your head, begin the chest press. Slowly lower the dumbbells to bring your forearms to rest flat on the floor. Keep the weights level as you bring your elbows down toward the floor.

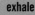 inhale ▶ exhale ▶ inhale **11**

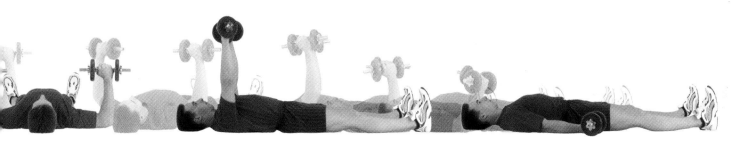

● Hold the weights so that your palms are facing down toward your feet. Your elbows, hands, and arms should be pointing upright toward the sky, with your palms facing down toward your feet.

● Inhale and slowly raise the weights in a vertical movement. Bring the weights together so that your arms are locked at the elbows and pointing toward the sky. Again, you will feel a contraction in your chest as you push upward.

● Lower the weights back down to the floor, then repeat the movement without straining the muscles. When you have finished a number of repetitions, bring your arms to your sides and relax.

● In both movements, all the weight is centered on the shoulders and upper back. For safety, if you feel any back strain, try doing the exercise with your knees raised and your feet flat on the floor.

exhale ▶ **inhale** ▶ **exhale** ▶ **breathe normally** ■

one arm dumbbell row

latissimus dorsi and biceps

This exercise mainly works the latissimus dorsi muscles, but also give the biceps and posterior shoulder muscles a workout. In order to isolate the latissimus dorsi muscles, correct posture is essential when performing this movement.

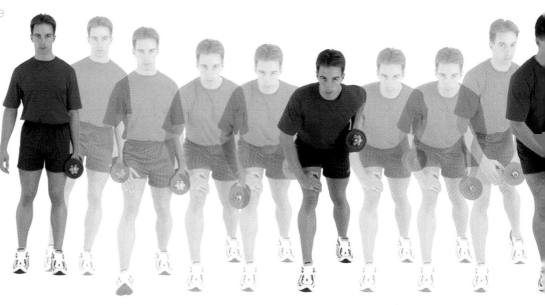

● Begin by stepping your left foot back about 24 inches (60 centimeters). Rest your right hand just above the flexed knee and lean forward. This will support your body weight and help maintain balance.

● Keeping your back straight and your shoulders and hips level and square, let the weight of the dumbbell pull your arm into position. Now lift your elbow and pull the weight up toward your chest.

● Raise the dumbbell until your elbow is in line with your shoulder. You will feel a contraction in the biceps and latissimus dorsi. Keep your shoulders level and do not twist the body as you lift, as this will bring into play a different group of muscles.

■   **inhale**   ▶   **begin to exhale**   ▶   **exhale**   ▶

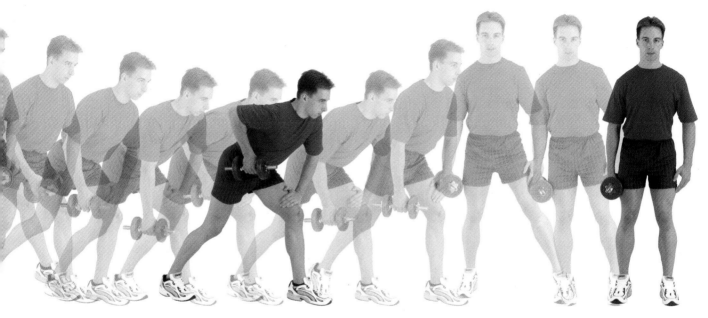

● Lower the dumbbell back to the starting position, keeping your hips and shoulders square. Repeat the movement without straining.

● Now switch the dumbbell to the other hand, stepping your right leg back and resting your left hand on your flexed left knee. Let the weight of the dumbbell pull your arm into position. Now pull the weight up toward your chest.

● Raise the dumbbell until your elbow is roughly in line with your shoulder. You will feel a contraction in your latissimus dorsi. Remember to keep your hips and shoulders level and your back straight.

● Now lower the dumbbell and repeat the exercise without straining. When you have finished, return to standing upright, with your back straight, your feet shoulder width apart and your hands at your sides.

❙❙   **inhale**   ▶   **exhale**   ▶   **breathe normally**   ■

shoulder retraction and reverse raise

The shoulder retraction will
work your upper back and
rear shoulder (rhomboid and
posterior deltoids) muscles,
while the reverse raise will test
the posterior deltoids
and the triceps.

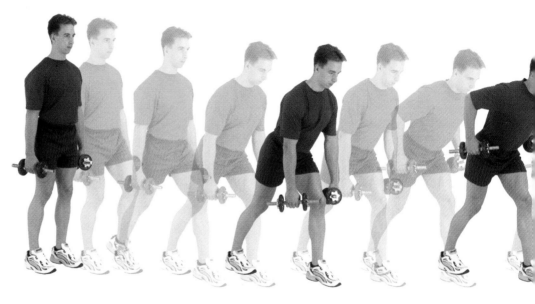

● Step one foot back 24 inches
(60 centimeters). Keep your back
straight and your shoulders and hips
level. Flex from the waist. Let the
dumbbells pull your arms into
position.

● Now perform the shoulder
retraction. To begin the move, retract
the shoulders. Keep the trunk of your
body stable and firm—all the movement
should be in the shoulders and arms.
Keep your back straight and shoulders
and hips square.

● Now pull both arms up and toward
the chest, bringing your elbows up to an
angle of 90 degrees. Hold the pose
briefly before lowering the dumbbells.
Repeat the exercise without straining
your muscles.

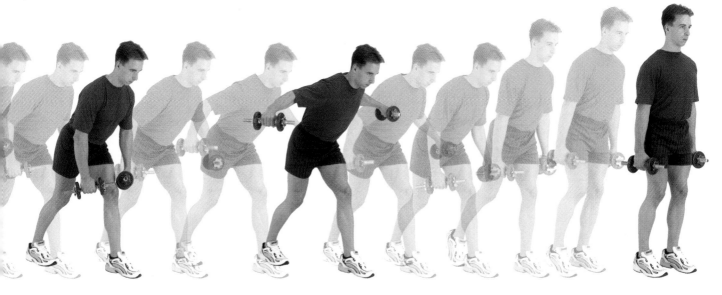

● Now prepare to perform the reverse raise. Retaining the same leg positions, let the gravitational pull of the dumbbells bring your arms into position, with hands suspended next to your knees.

● Now slowly lift your arms out to the sides, keeping the palms facing downward. Pull the dumbbells outward until they are in line with your chest, keeping the hands aligned.

● You will feel a contraction in your shoulders and in the rhomboid muscles between your shoulder blades. Only lift as far as it feels comfortable to do so. Hold the pose briefly, then repeat the lift without straining your muscles.

● Now release the pose, bring your feet back together, and return to standing upright with the dumbbells resting at your sides.

inhale ▶ **begin to exhale** ▶ **exhale** ▶ **breathe normally** ■

anterior and lateral raises

This sequence consists of two exercises that will work the anterior and medial deltoid muscles in the shoulders. The trapezius muscle in your upper back and neck will perform a stabilizing role.

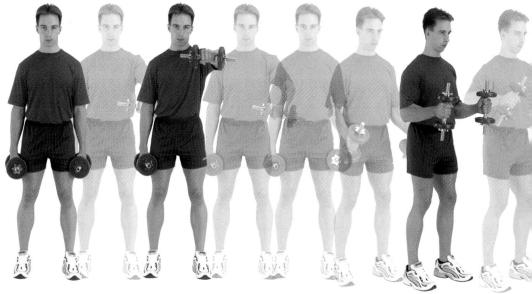

● Begin the exercise by exhaling and slowly raising your left arm, flexing at the shoulder to 90 degrees, with the elbow soft. Remember not to roll your body back as you raise the weight—all the movement should be isolated in the shoulder.

● As you raise your arm, slowly revolve the wrist 90 degrees so that your palm is facing downward, to rotate the dumbbell. Hold the pose for a second. Now lower the dumbbell back to the resting position. Repeat the raise without straining.

● To perform the lateral raise, bring the dumbbells in front of your chest so that your elbows are flexed to 90 degrees and the palms of your hands are facing inward. You should lift from the shoulders, and not merely raise your hands.

| ▪ | inhale | begin to exhale | ▶ | exhale | ‖ | inhale | ▶ |

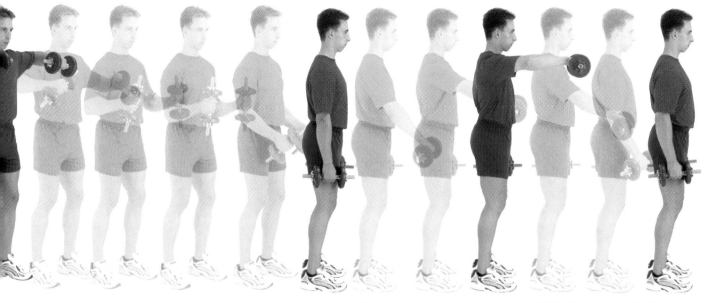

● From this starting position, raise the dumbbells. Imagine you are lifting your elbows at your sides but at the same time pointing your forearms forward in front of you in a curling motion. Move them up to shoulder height until your arms are parallel with the floor.

● Your hands should be the same height as your elbows to gain the full raise. Hold the pose briefly. Now lower the weights and repeat the lateral raise, remembering to keep your elbows aligned throughout.

● Now perform the single arm anterior raise with your right arm. Exhale and raise your right arm, flexing at the shoulder to 90 degrees. Remember not to roll your body back as you raise the weight.

● Now lower the dumbbell back to the resting position. Repeat the raise on the opposite arm without straining.

begin to exhale ▶ exhale ❚❚ exhale ▶ inhale ■

shrugs and upright row *trapezius and deltoids*

These two movements will work the trapezius muscle in the upper back and neck, and to a lesser extent, the deltoid muscles in the shoulders. Throughout this sequence it is important to hold a steady posture and keep the knees soft to maintain balance.

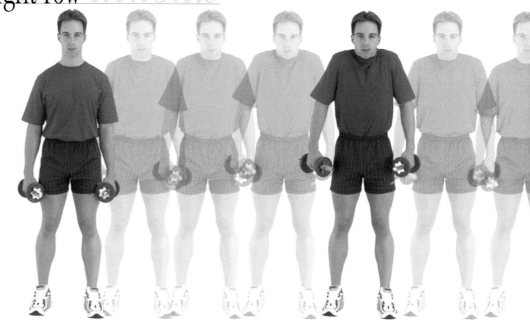

● Hold the weights at your sides, letting gravity pull them into position. Face forward with your head up. Exhale and shrug both shoulders together, lifting them toward your ears.

● Elevate your shoulders but do not rotate them. Hold this pose for a second. Now inhale and drop your shoulders back to the start position. Repeat the exercise without straining your muscles.

● Bring your shoulders back to a normal resting position and relax. From the same position, you can perform the upright row.

begin to exhale ▶ **exhale** ‖ **inhale** ▶

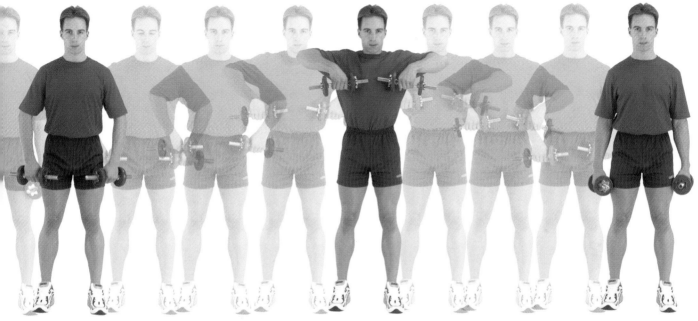

● To begin the exercise, raise your elbows upward and out to your sides. The dumbbells should remain below the level of your elbows—let your body guide you. Bring the elbows as high as possible, but keeping your hands down.

● Avoid hyperextending the spine by leaning back—keep your back straight and your body relaxed throughout the movement. All the movement should be in the shoulders and neck. Hold the pose for a second.

● Lower the dumbbells back to the start position, keeping your knuckles pointed downward throughout the movement. Repeat the raise without straining your muscles.

● Now bring the dumbbells back to your sides. Rest your shoulders and breathe deeply to relax.

begin to exhale ▶ **exhale** ‖ **inhale** ▶ **exhale** ■

concentration curl with hammer

These exercises work the biceps and the brachioradialis muscle in the lower arm. The concentration curl will make the biceps more prominent, while the hammer curl will thicken the muscle.

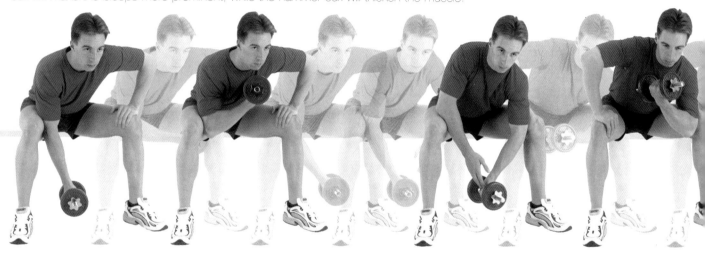

● The concentration curl is designed to isolate and work the biceps. To set up, sit on a chair, with your feet spaced 24 inches (60 centimeters) apart. Lean forward from the waist, keeping your back straight and your shoulders square.

● Holding the dumbbell, let your right hand drop down so that your triceps press against your right inner thigh. Your thigh should act as a pivot point for your arm. Rest the other hand on the left knee to provide support for your body weight.

● Hold the dumbbell with your palm facing outward. Slowly raise the weight, flexing at the elbow and contracting your biceps. Make sure your triceps remain pressed into the inner thigh—do not lean your body back to help pull up the weight.

● Now lower the dumbbell to the start position. You will feel a stretch in your biceps. Repeat the exercise without straining. Now switch the dumbbell to your left hand and perform the lift on the other side.

■ **begin to inhale** ▶ **inhale** ▶ **exhale** ❙❙ **inhale** ▶

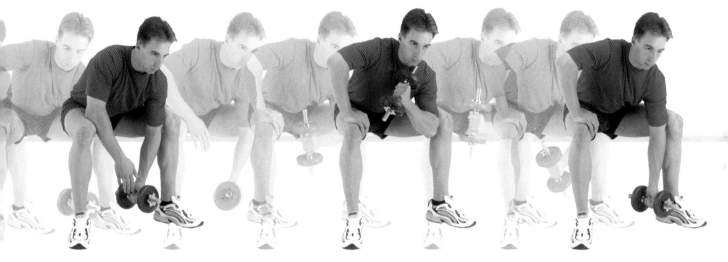

● To perform the hammer curl, use the same set up position, holding the dumbbell in your left hand. Sit on the chair and lean forward, keeping your back straight and your shoulders level.

● Press your triceps into your left inner thigh. This time, rotate your wrist so that your knuckles are in line with your forearm and your palm faces in. Holding the dumbbell at this angle will allow you to contract the brachioradialis to thicken the biceps.

● Now lift your arm, flexing at the elbow, bringing the dumbbell up so that the end is pointing toward your shoulder. Keep your triceps pressed firmly against the thigh. As you lift the weight, the brachioradialis muscle in the forearm will become more prominent.

● Now lower the dumbbell and return to the start position. Repeat the exercise without straining. Now perform the lift using the other arm.

‖ inhale ▶ begin to exhale ▶ exhale ▶ inhale ‖

standing triceps kickback with biceps curl

These two exercises will test your triceps and biceps. The triceps kickback is a difficult exercise and should only be attempted after doing plenty of basic exercises to improve coordination.

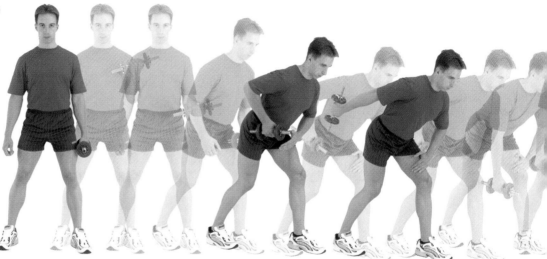

● To set up for the tricep kickback, step the right foot backward to get into a low position. Lean forward and place your resting hand just in front of your flexed knee for stability. Keep your back straight and your shoulders square.

● Now lift your right elbow to bring it level with the floor, keeping your upper arm rigid but letting your lower arm hang loose. Your extended upper arm must remain stable throughout the exercise. You are now ready to perform the triceps extension.

● Extending from the elbow, raise your forearm to extend the arm fully and lock the elbow. Remember not to twist or rotate your body when raising your arm. Now lower your arm and return to standing upright with your feet spaced apart.

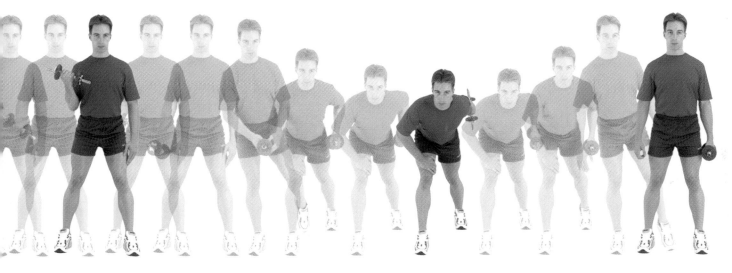

● To set up for the biceps curl, flex your triceps and latissimus dorsi muscles to provide stability. This will ensure that all the focus is concentrated on the biceps. Do not press your elbows into your sides, as this will reduce the effectiveness.

● Exhale and slowly lift the dumbbell toward your shoulders. Stop when the biceps are fully flexed. Do not try to raise the dumbbell any further, as this will cause the elbow to move and start to contract the shoulders.

● Inhale and lower the dumbbell back to the start position. Repeat the curls without straining. Now step your right foot forward in order to set up for the tricep kickback with the left arm.

● Perform the tricep extension with your left arm, repeating without straining the muscle. Now repeat the biceps curl using your left arm. When you have finished, return to the upright standing position and relax.

inhale ▶ exhale ▶ inhale ❙❙ inhale ▶ exhale ■

french press with overhead raise

triceps and latissimus dorsi

This is a more difficult sequence that will work your triceps and latissimus dorsi muscles. The French press can be performed either one arm at a time or both together.

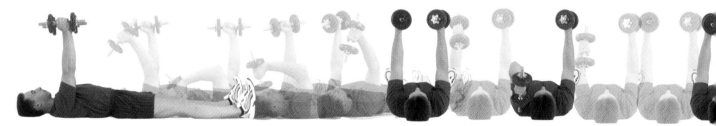

● Lie on your back with your legs extended and your feet spaced evenly apart. Raise the dumbbells above your chest, extending your arms fully but soft at the elbows. You are now ready to perform the French press.

● Flexing from the elbow, lower the right dumbbell toward your head to bring your forearm approximately parallel with the floor. Aim for a 90 degree flexion at the elbow.

● Now raise the dumbbell back to the start position. You will feel pressure on your right triceps. The upper arm should remain stable throughout the movement in order to isolate and work the triceps.

● Now perform the exercise using the other arm, flexing from the elbow. Repeat the press with both arms, remembering not to over strain the tricep muscles. Advanced exercisers can perform the movement using both arms at once.

■   inhale   ▶   exhale   ▶   inhale   ▶   exhale

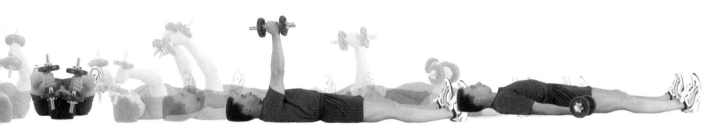

● Now return both dumbbells to the start position, raised above your chest with your arms fully extended. Keeping your arms fully extended, lower both dumbbells behind your head. You are ready to perform the overhead raise.

● Flexing from the shoulders, raise the dumbbells over your head, keeping your arms fully extended throughout the movement. Lift the dumbbells until you have returned to the start position.

● You will feel a contraction in your latissimus dorsi muscles and triceps. Repeat either exercise to concentrate the focus on a specific muscle.

● Once you have completed the necessary number of repetitions, lower the dumbbells to your sides, breathe deeply and relax.

|| inhale   ▶   exhale   ▶   inhale   ▶   exhale   ■

exercise ball

ball squat and single leg

quadriceps and gluteus maximus

This exercise will improve your core stability and work the quadricep muscles at the front of the thighs and the gluteal muscles in the buttocks.

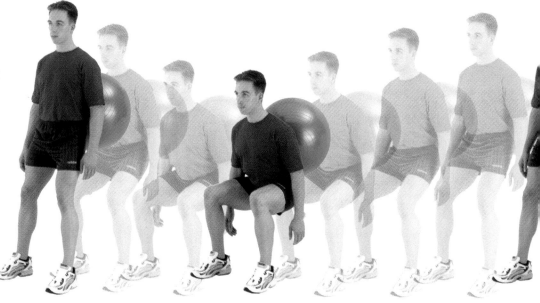

● To set up, begin by trapping the ball between yourself and the wall, with the ball tucked in the small of your back. Your legs should be slightly bent at the knees. Keep your arms relaxed at your sides.

● Slowly lower your body, flexing the knees to 90 degrees. Roll your body down the ball. Finish this movement with the ball pressed between your shoulder blades. Your bottom should be slightly under the ball.

● To gain the maximum resistance, keep your body pressed tightly against the ball. Now raise yourself back up to the start position. Throughout the movement you will feel a contraction in the quadriceps.

exhale ▶ inhale ▶ exhale

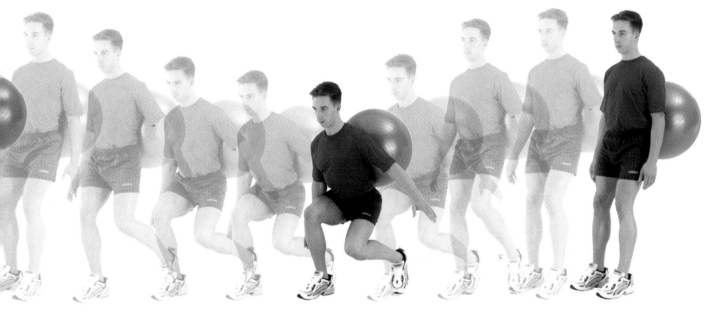

● Now return to the start position. To do the single leg advanced version, squat on one leg, using the resting foot to help you maintain balance. The balancing leg should not be taking any of the weight, but should stop your body from swiveling out of position.

● Now inhale and slowly dip down. When fully depressed, your right knee should remain in line with your foot and not be extended further forward than your toes. Your back will roll beneath the ball. Use your left arm to help maintain balance.

● Exhale as you rise to the start position. Feel the pressure on your quadriceps as you dip, and on your gluteal muscles as you rise again. Keep your hips square to stop your body rolling around the ball. Repeat the exercise without straining.

● Now perform the exercise with the other leg. As a further progression, you can hold dumbbells to increase the weight. If you wish to tone the insides of your thighs, perform the squats with your feet spread more widely apart.

begin to inhale   ▶   **inhale**   ▶   **exhale**   ▶   ■

lying hamstrings curl and single leg

hamstrings and gluteus maximus

This is an advanced exercise that will work your hamstrings and the gluteal muscles in your buttocks. For this routine, your torso and abdomen must be strong to act as stabilizing muscles.

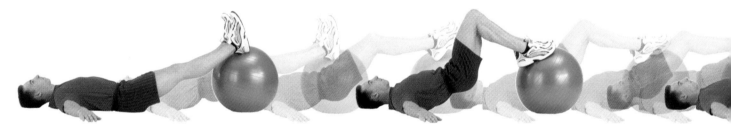

● To set up, lie on the floor with your arms extended flat and your fingers splayed out to provide support. With knees bent, rest the soles of your feet on the top of the ball.

● Now extend your legs to lock at the knees so that your heels are resting on the ball. Tense your gluteal muscles. Your body should be straight and rigid, from your lower back to your heels. You are now ready to begin the hamstring curl.

● To begin the exercise, bring your knees back toward your head, rolling the ball beneath your feet. Keep your lower back, gluteal muscles and hips rigid to maintain balance. You can also push with your arms against the floor to maintain pressure.

● Complete the rolling motion until the soles of your feet are flat against the ball. Your knees should form an angle of 90 degrees. Now roll the ball back under your feet and fully extend your legs to return to the start position. Repeat the exercise without straining.

inhale ▶ **exhale** ▶ **inhale** **11**

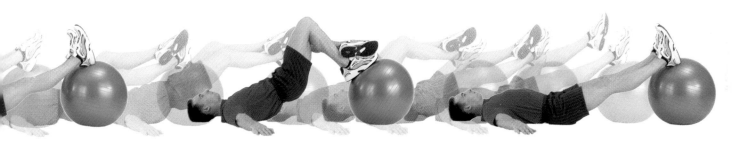

● To do a single leg variation, rest the passive foot over the shin of the active foot. All the weight is then concentrated on one leg. This is an advanced exercise that only those with very good abdominal strength should consider.

● As with the two-legged version, bring your knee back toward your head, rolling the ball beneath your foot. Keep your lower back, gluteals and hips rigid. Push with your arms against the floor to maintain pressure.

● Again, bring the leg back until the knee forms a 90 degree angle. Now roll the ball back under your foot and fully extend your leg to return to the start position. For an effective posture, throughout the movement you will need to keep your hips square.

● Repeat the exercise without straining, then perform the movement with the other leg. Once you have finished repeating the exercises, return your legs to the start position and relax.

inhale   ▶   **exhale**   ▶   **inhale**   ▶   **breathe normally**   ■

gluteal raise *maximus*

This is a beginner's exercise that will work and strengthen your gluteal muscles. It is very important to keep your hips in the correct posture when performing this exercise.

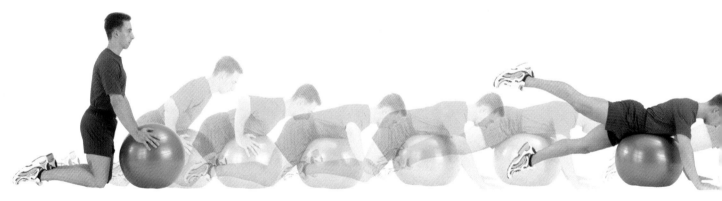

- To set up, kneel on the floor and place the ball in front of your knees. Grip the ball with your hands and lean forward to bring your chest down to rest on the top of the ball.

- Roll the ball beneath your body until your abdomen is resting on the ball and your extended legs are balancing on the tips of your toes. Press the palms of your hands flat on the floor to maintain balance.

- To begin the exercise, exhale and raise your extended right leg vertically as high as possible. (This will depend on individual flexibility—only raise your leg as far as it feels comfortable.)

- As you raise your leg, remember to push down with your hands to help maintain balance and stability. You will feel a contraction in your right gluteal muscles. Hold the position briefly.

inhale   ▶   **begin to exhale**   ▶   **exhale**   ▶

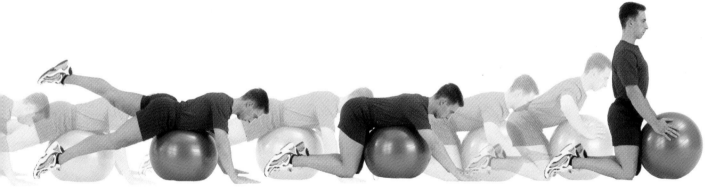

● Now inhale and lower your leg to the start position. Repeat the exercise with the left leg. Exhale and raise your extended left leg vertically as high as you can while keeping your hips square and aligned.

● When lifting your leg, do not try to raise it too far—your hips should not leave the surface of the ball, otherwise your body will begin to twist, putting your lower back under strain. Repeat the raise without straining the muscles.

● Now release the position and roll the ball beneath your chest to bring your knees to rest on the floor.

● Lift your body away from the ball and return to the kneeling upright position. Breathe deeply and relax.

inhale   ‖   **begin to exhale**   **exhale**   ▶   **inhale**   ▶   **exhale**   ■

lying hip flexor

This exercise works your hip flexors and abdominal muscles and will test your core stability to the full. Although this exercise concentrates on the lower torso, it also requires good upper body strength to hold the body in position.

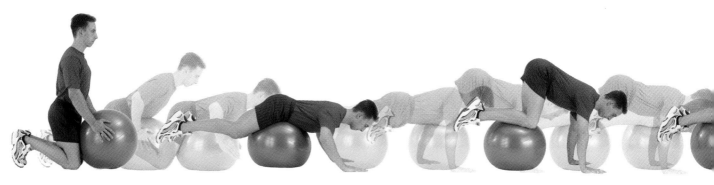

● Kneel behind the ball and grip it firmly at the sides. Lean forward and roll your body over the ball. Move to bring the ball beneath your abdomen.

● Now place your hands on the floor. Slowly walk your hands forward until the ball is positioned beneath your thighs. Your hands and feet should be spaced as widely apart as possible to help you maintain balance.

● To begin the exercise, raise your hips and bottom and roll the ball under your knees, while keeping your back straight and your elbows soft. Your shoulders and arms will hold your body in position. The movement should come from the legs and hips.

● Continue the movement until your knees form a 90 degree angle and the ball is beneath your shins. Remember to only move to the point where your back can remain rigid—otherwise your back will arch and you may lose balance. Return to the start position.

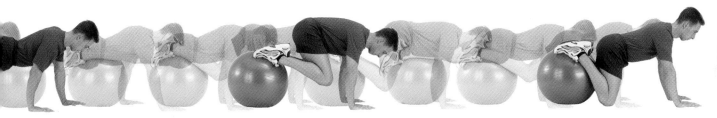

● If you have the necessary abdominal strength, you can begin a second, more advanced move from this position. Slowly walk forward on your arms so that your legs are fully extended and your shins are resting on the ball.

● Now progress the move, raising your bottom by flexing from the hips. Remember to only flex to the point where your back is still rigid.

● You should be able to flex to the point where the tops of your feet are resting on the ball. You will feel a lot of pressure on your abdominal muscles and in your hips. Hold this pose briefly, then roll your feet back to bring your knees to rest on the floor.

● Repeat both variations as many times as possible without causing muscle strain.

inhale ▶ **exhale** ▶ **inhale** ▶ **exhale** ❙❙

standing calf raise
gastrocnemius muscle

This exercise will work your calf muscles. The ball provides compression and additional friction to increase the resistance. You will need a shallow step or platform close to a wall to be able to perform this routine.

- To set up, stand facing away from the wall, with the ball balanced in the small of your back. Rest your feet on a shelf or step about two inches (five centimeters) deep.

- To begin the movement, exhale and slowly lift yourself by plantarflexing on the balls of your feet, rolling your body up the ball. To increase the resistance, remember to press your back into the ball throughout the exercise.

- As you raise yourself from the calves, also lift up your arms while keeping your palms flat and facing downward. This will help you balance on the balls of your feet. Keep your knees locked throughout the movement.

- Now inhale and gently lower yourself back to the start position. Note that only a little movement is needed to exercise the calves, and the ball does not move very far. Repeat the exercise without straining.

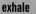

begin to exhale ▶ exhale ▶ inhale

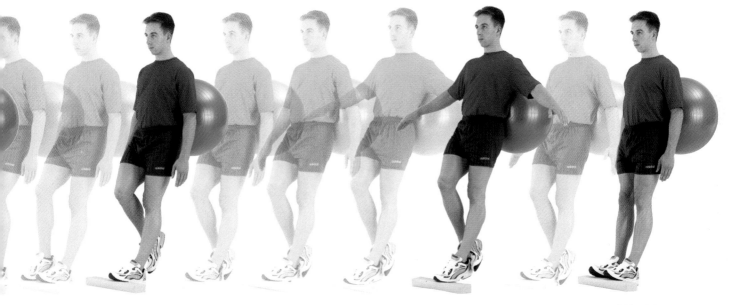

● To do a single leg variation, rest the passive foot behind your active heel, but without touching the floor. All the weight should be concentrated on your working foot.

● Exhale and slowly lift yourself by plantarflexing on the ball of your foot, rolling your body up the ball. Keep your knee locked throughout the movement in order to concentrate all the pressure on the calf muscles.

● Now inhale and gently lower yourself back to the start position. Repeat the calf raise without causing a muscle strain. Now perform the raise on the other leg.

● When you have finished the repetitions, rest your heels on the floor and bring your arms to your sides. Relax and breathe deeply.

inhale ▶ exhale ▶ inhale ▶ exhale ■

stability press ups *triceps and deltoids*

This routine works the chest, triceps, and shoulder muscles. Good torso strength

is required to stabilize the body. Beginners should only try the kneeling variation.

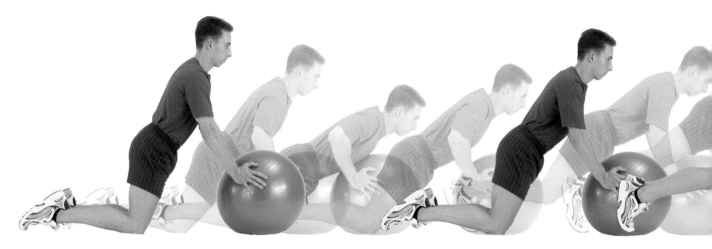

● To set up, kneel behind the ball. Rest your hands on the front of the ball and grip the ridges to avoid straining your wrists. Your toes should be curled to touch the floor and help you maintain balance.

● Now lean forward, taking your upper body weight on your arms, with your chest resting on the ball. It is important that your torso remains rigid throughout the movement.

● To begin the exercise, exhale and lift yourself from the ball, keeping your body rigid and flexing from the knees. All the movement should be concentrated in your triceps and chest, where you will feel pressure.

● Now lower yourself back down toward the ball. Repeat a number of dips until you are tired. Remember that you should be dipping your whole body from the waist upward, and not just your chest and shoulders.

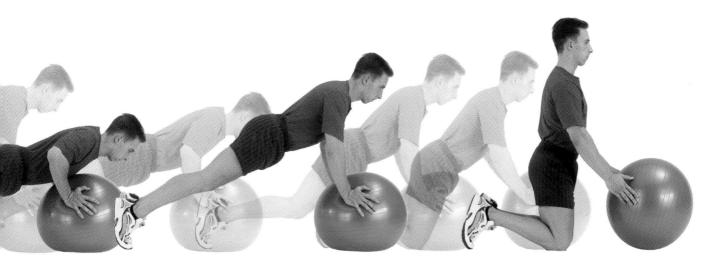

● Those with good torso and arm strength can try the advanced version. To set up, extend your legs to lock at the knees so that you are balancing on your toes. Make your body rigid, with your chest resting on the ball. Grip the ball with your chest resting on the top.

● Now perform the lifts and dips, keeping your body rigid throughout. All the movement should be concentrated in your triceps and chest, where you will feel a great deal of pressure.

● Remember to exhale as you push upward and inhale as you lower yourself toward the ball. Repeat the press ups as many times as you can without causing a strain in your back, abdomen or arms.

● Now bring your knees back down to the floor, raise your body to kneel upright and relax.

inhale ▶ **exhale** ▶ **inhale** ▶ **exhale** ■

stability push downs

latissimus dorsi and pectoralis

This exercise will work your back and chest muscles—the latissimus dorsi and pectoralis. There are two versions, a beginner's and an advanced, but only those with good torso strength should attempt the advanced routine.

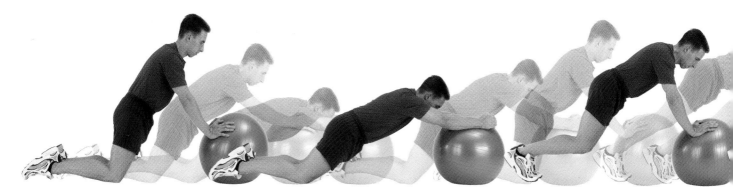

● To set up, kneel behind the ball, resting your hands on the front and gripping the ridges to avoid straining your wrists. Your hands should be evenly spaced for good balance.

● To begin the exercise, inhale and slowly lower your body forward, rolling the ball under your hands, wrists, and forearms in a smooth steady movement. Keep your back rigid as you move forward.

● Your legs should be relaxed, providing support from the knees. Fully extend this pose as far as you can without toppling over. At full stretch, your bottom should remain in line with your back. You will feel a contration in your latissimus dorsi.

● Remember to only roll as far as you feel comfortable—if your abdominal and lower back muscles begin to feel strained, stop the exercise. Now exhale and roll back to the starting position.

| | begin to inhale | ▶ | inhale | ▶ | exhale | **11** |

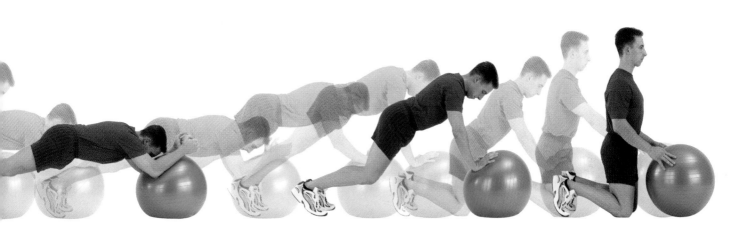

● Now perform the advanced variation. Roll the ball forward until you are balancing on your toes, with your whole body rigid. Keep your back straight, but not in a perfect line with your legs, as this will strain your body a great deal.

● Roll your body until your elbows are resting on the ball and your body is extended, balancing on your toes. Clasp your hands together to steady yourself. Hold the position briefly.

● Now return to the start position, rolling your body backward and pushing your body away from the ball to extend your arms. Unclasp your hands and bring the palms to rest on the ball.

● Flexing at the knees, lower your legs down to the floor and bring your body upright. Relax your muscles and breathe deeply.

inhale ▶ **inhale** ▶ **exhale** ▶ **breathe normally** ■

stability dips *and anterior deltoids*

This is an advanced exercise that will challenge your core stability

and work your triceps, shoulders, and anterior deltoids.

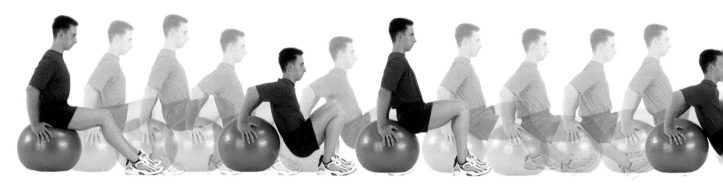

● To set up, sit upright on the center of the ball, with your feet flat on the floor. Grip the ball at the sides to provide support for your wrists. Your hands should be evenly spaced to maintain balance and avoid the ball twisting out of position.

● Begin the exercise by slowly shifting your weight forward. Lower yourself but without resting your body on the ball. All the movement should be in the elbow joints—your torso and hips should remain taut and aligned.

● Lower your body until your upper arms are roughly parallel to the floor. Now push upward while maintaining your balance. At this point you will feel the most strain on your triceps and shoulders.

● Continue to push upward, while maintaining your balance and keeping your torso straight. All the movement should be in your elbows. Return to the start position, sitting on the ball.

■ inhale ▶ exhale ▶ inhale **11**

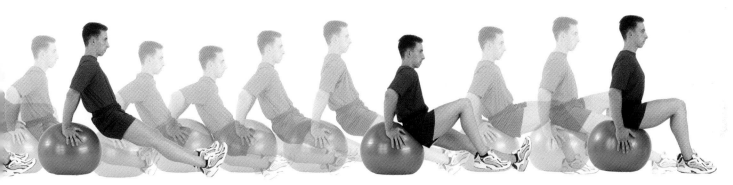

● This second movement is only for those with good upper body strength. Sit slightly further forward on the ball. Grip the ball just behind your hips and balance your body on your heels. You will need to keep your legs locked at the knees to maintain balance.

● Now lower yourself again, keeping your body straight and bearing your weight on your arms. This exercise will put extra strain on the triceps and shoulders. Lower yourself only as far as it feels comfortable.

● Now raise your body by pushing upward with your arms. Fully extend your arms and hold yourself with elbows locked. Now gently lower yourself and return to the seated start position.

● Repeat the stability dips as many times as you can without causing muscle strain. Afterward, sit upright on the ball and relax your muscles.

exhale ▶ **inhale** ▶ **exhale** ▶ ∎

lower back raise

This is a difficult exercise that will challenge your core stability. Do not attempt this exercise if you have recently suffered an injury to your lower back.

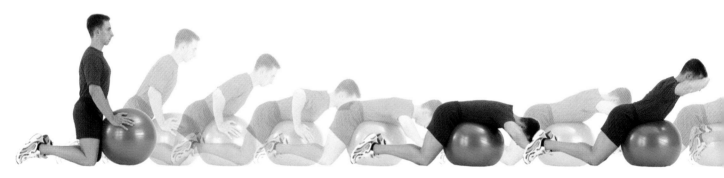

● To set up, kneel behind the ball, gripping the ridges to avoid putting pressure on your wrists. Now lean forward over the ball, keeping your knees on the floor.

● Walk your hands forward until your abdomen is resting on the top of the ball and your thighs are pressed against the front of the ball. Your knees should be pressed on the floor to provide stability for the exercise.

● To begin the exercise, rest the backs of your hands against your forehead. Your hands are there to support your head so that you do not strain your neck muscles, which should be relaxed throughout the movement.

● Now exhale and slowly lift your upper body from the abdomen. Raise your body as high as possible without straining. Push from the feet to provide lift and maintain tension. You will feel a stretch in your lower back.

■　　　▶　　　inhale　　　▶　　　exhale　　　▶

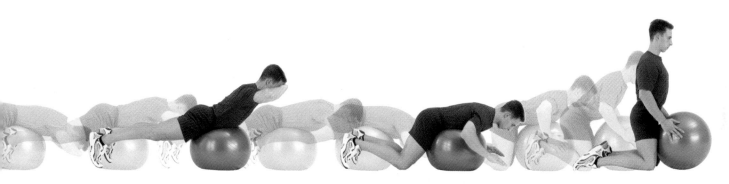

● Now inhale and lower your torso back to the start position. Remember to keep your neck relaxed throughout the movement. Repeat the movement as many times as possible without straining the muscles.

● To set up for the more difficult variation, extend your legs backward to bring your knees off the floor. Balance on your toes with your abdomen resting on the ball.

● Exhale and repeat the movement, lifting your upper body as high as you can. Do not let your feet leave the floor, or you may become unbalanced.

● Now inhale and lower yourself back to the start position. Lift your body away from the ball and return to the upright kneeling position. Relax your muscles and breathe deeply.

inhale   ❚❚   **begin to exhale**   ▶   **exhale**   ▶   **inhale**   ■

ball crunch *inals*

This is an advanced exercise that will give your abdominal muscles a good

workout. Using the ball for this movement provides extra stability while

reducing the risk of injury to your abdomen.

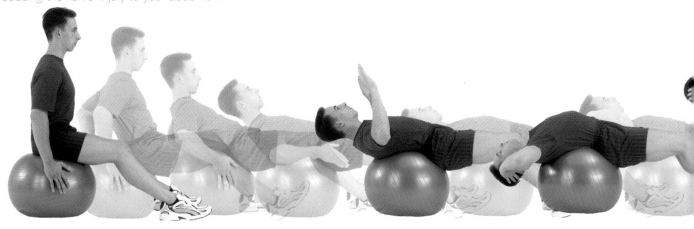

● The exercise ball is an excellent tool for performing abdominal crunches, as it allows you to lower your body below the midline while providing solid and flexible support for a more extreme abdominal workout.

● Begin the movement sitting on the exercise ball with your hands resting at your sides. To set up, slowly roll your body over the ball, walking your feet forward to bring the small of your back to rest on the top of the ball.

● Press your feet flat against the floor, with your knees locked for stability and balance. Place your hands behind your head to provide support for the neck.

● Now raise your upper body, flexing from the abdomen. Try not to tense your neck muscles—all the movement should come from the stomach, and only the abdominal muscles should be working.

■   **inhale**   ▶   **begin to exhale**   ▶   **exhale**   ▶

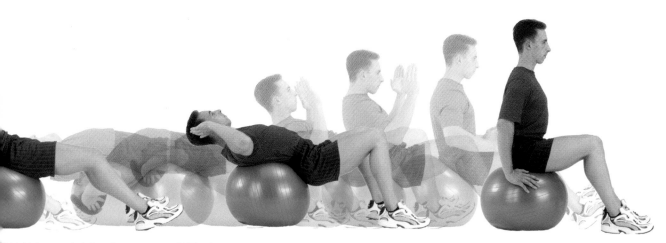

● Hold the pose briefly, trying not to tense your neck muscles. Remember to keep your thighs level and knees locked throughout the crunch to provide a solid foundation for the movement.

● Now lower your head back toward the floor, lowering your body as far as it feels comfortable to do so. This counterpose will help stretch the abdominal muscles in the opposing direction and release muscle tension.

● Allow gravity to take your body down as far as possible, but without becoming unbalanced. This will allow you to begin from a lower and more difficult position when repeating the abdominal crunch.

● Now repeat the crunches as many times as possible. When you have finished, lift yourself up and sit upright on the ball. Relax your muscles and breathe deeply. You can increase the intensity by positioning your body further back over the ball.

begin to inhale ▶ inhale ▶ exhale ▶ breathe normally ■

core stability

ball plank

obliques and abdominals

This is an advanced exercise that will improve your core stability and work the inner muscles around the torso—the transversus abdominis, rectus abdominis, and internal and external obliques.

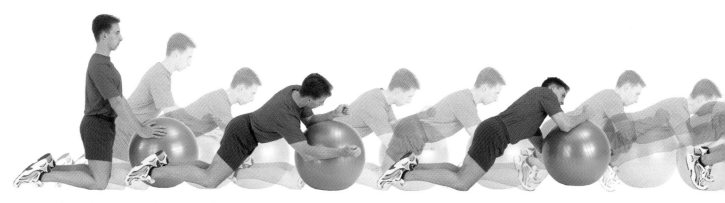

● This is a static movement where balance and correct positioning are crucial. This exercise will require constant breathing since the pose can be held for up to a minute. To set up, kneel behind the ball and place your hands on either side.

● To get into the start position, push your arms out, and roll the ball forward beneath your hands to rest your forearms on the top of the ball. Do not extend your arms too far, or your back will become arched. Keep your knees firmly on the floor.

● Keeping your back straight and your knees steady, roll your body to the right. Hold the pose for as long as you can. You will feel a contraction in the muscles around your abdomen and the sides of your torso.

● Now roll your body to the left and hold the pose. Only roll your body as far as you can while maintaining balance. Remember that your arms and shoulders should not be bearing the weight, but are there to provide stability. Release the pose and relax.

■   **inhale and exhale**   II   **inhale and exhale**   II   ▶

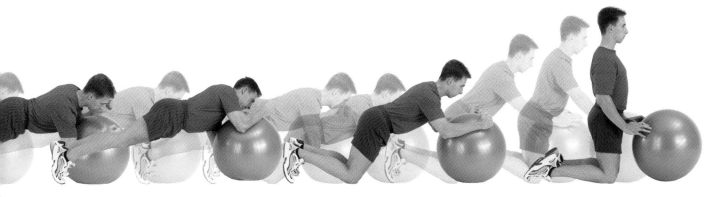

● To do a more advanced version, lift your knees from the floor and balance on your toes with your legs extended. As before, rest your forearms on the ball. Your legs and back should not form a straight line, as this will put too much strain on your back.

● Now do the rolls to the right and left, holding each pose for as long as you can without straining. This is a very difficult exercise, and you may find that you cannot hold the pose for as long as the earlier variation.

● Perform both variations as many times as you can without causing strain to your muscles.

● Now release the pose, bring your knees down to the floor and relax your muscles. Lift yourself away from the ball and kneel upright.

inhale and exhale　　‖　　inhale and exhale　　‖　　inhale　　▶　　exhale　　■

reverse ball plank *transversus abdominis*

This exercise will work all the inner muscles of your torso and lower back—the transversus abdominis, quadratus lumborum, rectus abdominis, and internal and external obliques.

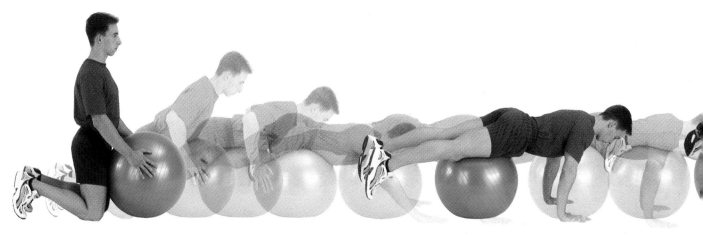

● Like the Ball plank sequence (see pages 66–67), this is a static movement where balancing and stability are crucial. Breathe deeply throughout the exercise—this will help you hold the pose more effectively.

● To set up, kneel behind the ball. Lean forward over the ball and place your hands flat on the floor. Now walk your hands forward until your thighs are resting on the top of the ball. Make sure your elbows and shoulders are soft.

● To begin the exercise, slowly roll your thighs to the right while maintaining good balance. Keep your feet out wide and your hands pressed firmly on the floor. Hold the pose.

● Now roll in the opposite direction and hold the pose. Only roll as far as you can without affecting your balance. Keep your back straight throughout to avoid sinking and straining your back muscles.

■   ▶   **inhale and exhale**   ‖   **inhale and exhale**   ‖

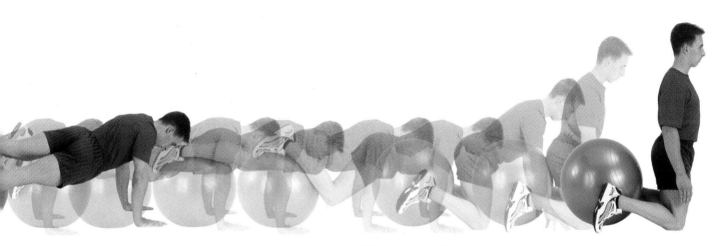

● The advanced version should only be attempted by those who have excellent allround body strength. To do this variation, walk forward on your hands so that your shins rest on the top of the ball. Space your legs wide for better balance.

● Now roll your shins to the right and then to the left, keeping your back rigid and your elbows and shoulders locked throughout. Hold the pose with each roll, remembering not to become unbalanced and without straining.

● This movement will put much more strain on the body, and requires a lot greater strength, balance, and stability.

● Now release the pose and relax your muscles, bringing your knees down to the floor to rest. Kneel upright and bring your hands to your sides. Breathe deeply and relax.

inhale and exhale   ❙❙   **inhale and exhale**   ❙❙   **inhale**   ▶   **exhale**   ◼

torso raise and press *and deltoids*

This series of exercises works and strengthens all your inner torso muscles—transversus abdominis, quadratus lumborum, rectus abdominis, and internal and external obliques—as well as your deltoids.

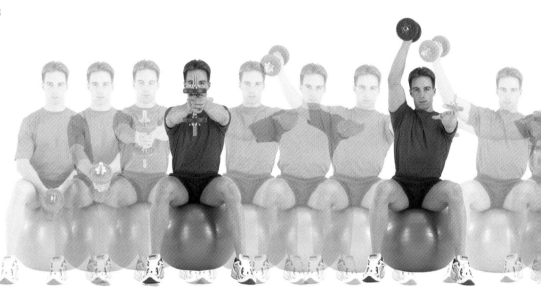

● Sit on the ball, with your feet on the floor, shoulder width apart. Using both hands, raise the dumbbell in front of you. Although you are using your arms and shoulder muscles, the ball moves all the stress to the torso by forcing the body to balance.

● Raise the dumbbell to roughly lower chest height and then hold it there for 30 seconds. Your torso will feel tight and taut. Remember to keep your hips square on the ball to avoid arching your back. Lower the dumbbell and relax.

● Then, with the dumbbell in your right hand, extend your arm out to the side and raise it slowly above your head. Your left arm should be extended in front of your body with the palm facing downward. Hold for 30 seconds.

| inhale | ▶ | exhale and inhale | ‖ | exhale and inhale | ‖ |

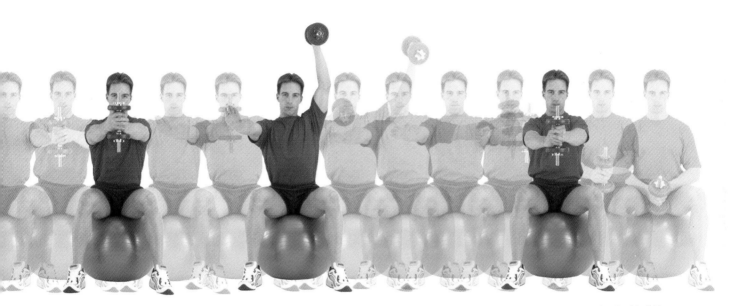

● Take the arm back down again and then repeat another dumbbell raise with both hands. Remember to only raise your arms to lower chest height. Again, hold the pose for 30 seconds to really contract the abdominal muscles.

● Now repeat the single arm movement with the dumbbell in your left hand raised above your head and your right arm extended in front of you. Hold this position for 30 seconds.

● Lower your left arm slowly to the floor and repeat the initial dumbbell raise with two hands. Remember to keep your back straight and your legs steady for support. Hold the pose for 30 seconds.

● Now lower the dumbbell. You can repeat the exercises as many times as possible to give your inner muscles a good workout.

exhale and inhale　　　　　　**exhale and inhale**　　　**exhale**　　　　　▶　　　　■

torso twist

Like the Torso raise and press (see pages 70–71), this exercise strengthens all the inner torso muscles—transversus abdominis, quadratus lumborum, rectus abdominis, and internal and external obliques—by twisting the body while holding a dumbbell.

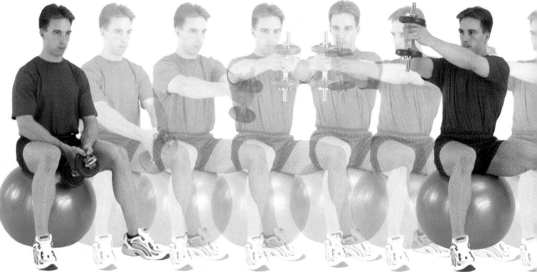

● Plant your feet roughly 14 inches (35 centimeters) apart. Using both hands, slowly raise the dumbbell and extend your arms out. The lift should come from your arms—don't lean your body back as you lift, as this will unbalance your posture.

● Now exhale and rotate your body to the right as far as it will go. The dumbbell should stay in line with your chin. Keep your legs still and supportive.

● Twist from the body and don't just move your arms. As you twist, turn your head to face toward the dumbbell. Your torso should feel tight and taut.

■　　　　　inhale　　　▶　　　exhale　　　　▶　　　inhale and exhale　　　▶

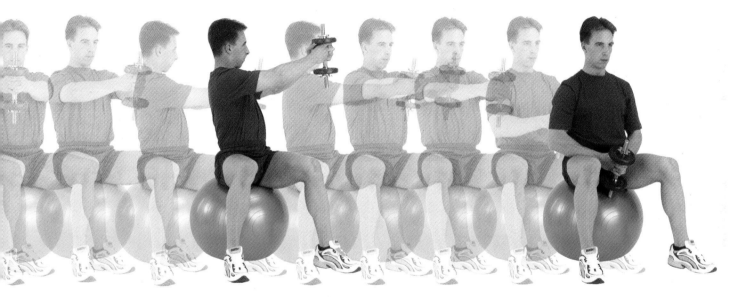

● Do not hold the pose, but inhale and move the dumbbell back to the start position. Remember to keep your hips square on the ball to avoid arching your back.

● Now do the exercise on the other side. Remember to twist from the waist and keep the dumbbell in line with your chin.

● As you twist and lift the dumbbell, make sure that you lift from the lower back but without leaning backward. This will work the muscles in your lower back.

● When you have finished the repetitions, lower the dumbbell carefully down to the start position and then relax.

inhale and exhale   ‖   ▶ **inhale and exhale**   **inhale and exhale**   ▶   ■

cable exercises

gluteal raise and kick *hamstrings*

This sequence works the front and back of the legs—the gluteal muscles and hamstrings. The exercise is divided into two parts, a gluteal raise and a more strenuous kickback. For both, you will need an ankle strap attachment.

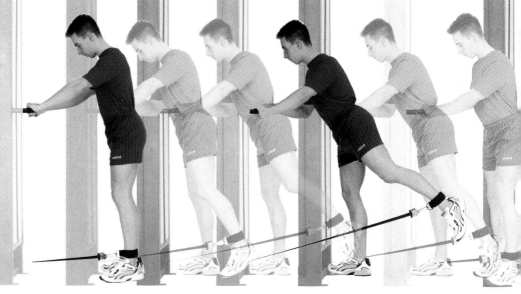

● Attach the ankle strap to your left ankle. Stand with both feet close together. Hold onto the bar for support. Now slowly lift and extend your left leg. Do not arch your back, and keep your abdominals tight to ensure your body remains stable.

● Keep raising your leg back as far as it will go without rotating your hips. Make sure you keep your hips square throughout the raise. Your standing leg should point outward slightly which will work the gluteals.

● Now slowly lower the leg back to the start position. Repeat the movement and then perform the exercise with your right leg.

| | inhale and exhale | ▶ | exhale | ▶ | inhale | ▶ |

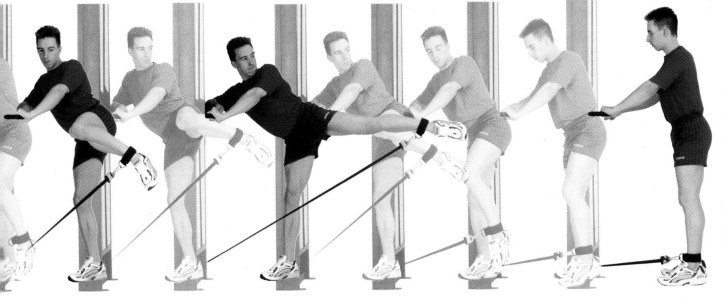

● To do the kickback variation, lean forward and balance your weight by holding on to the bar on the upright. To set up, start to raise your left leg so that it is parallel with the floor, forming a 90 degree angle with your standing leg. Your right knee should be soft.

● When raised, your leg will be bent at the knee. Now slowly extend your leg out in a kicking motion. Turn your head to face your left extended leg but be careful not to tense your shoulders.

● Fully extend your leg to reach waist height. Remember to keep your hips square; do not twist your body as you kick.

● Now bring your leg back so that it is bent at the knee, and kick out again. Do not rest your leg on the floor—all repetitions should be done while standing on one leg. Repeat the same exercise and repetitions with your right leg.

exhale ▶ inhale exhale ▶ ‖

adduction and abduction *gluteals*

These are two primary exercises for working the adductor muscles on the inside and outside of the thighs. For both variations you will need an ankle strap attachment.

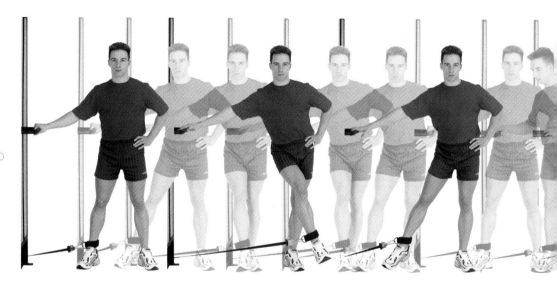

● To set up, stand with your feet about 15 inches (40 centimeters) apart. Stand close enough to the cable upright to hold onto the bar for support. Rest your other hand on your hip for balance.

● To perform the adduction, slowly draw your right foot inward across your other leg, as though passing a football with the inside of your foot. Extend the right leg as far as possible and lean slightly toward the machine.

● Keep your hips as square as possible. You will feel a contraction on the inside of your thigh. Now slowly return your foot to the start position. Repeat the movement, then do the exercise with the other leg.

inhale ▶ **exhale** ▶ **inhale** ▶

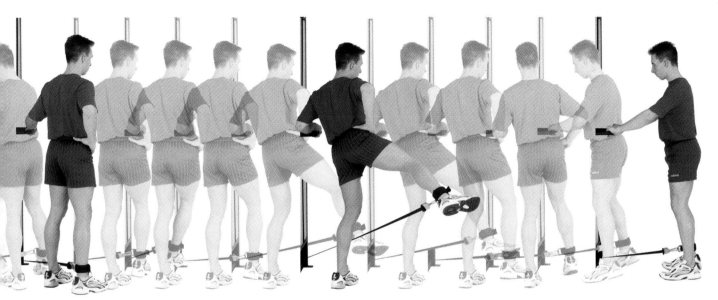

● To do the abduction, you will need to turn around, hold the bar with your left hand and bring the right leg over your left leg for the start position. Attach the cable and stand at a distance from the upright so that the cable is taut.

● Hold on to the bar on the column for balance, while resting your other hand on your hip. Take a breath in.

● Now gradually move your foot outward to work your gluteal muscles. Keep your standing foot steady and your hips square. Remain upright and try not to lean.

● Continue to raise your leg until it is roughly 45 degrees from the standing position. Hold briefly, then return to the start up position. Repeat the movement, then do the exercise with the other leg.

start to inhale   ▶   inhale   exhale   ▶   ❙❙

cable crossover *and deltoids*

This exercise will work and strengthen your pectoral muscles (chest) and your anterior deltoids (the front of the shoulders).

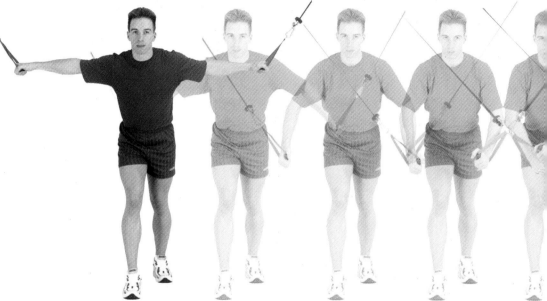

● Stand in the middle of the two cable uprights, slightly in front of center. Step forward with your right leg and lean to support your weight. Hold the handles with palms facing downward. Extend your arms out at right angles to your body.

● To begin the exercise, roll your arms toward each other, making sure that they remain roughly aligned throughout the movement. Remember to keep your abdominal muscles tight to provide support for your lower back.

● Continue extending your arms until your hands cross in the center to get a full contraction. All the resistance comes from behind the body, so you should concentrate on pushing forward and downward.

inhale ▶ **begin to exhale** ▶ **exhale** ▶

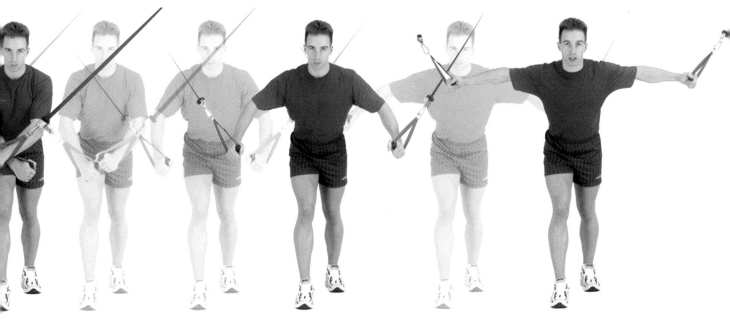

● Once your arms are fully flexed, you will feel a contraction in your shoulders and your chest, as well as a slight contraction in your biceps, which act as stabilizing muscles. Hold this position.

● Now take your arms back up again toward the ceiling. Keep your elbows slightly bent as you perform the move and make sure your torso and legs remain still and supportive.

● Take the arms back to the start position. Try not to hunch your shoulders as you move them. Remember to take your arms back to a 90 degree angle at the shoulder and no further.

● Repeat the exercise as many times as necessary, taking care not to strain your arm muscles and ensuring the movement is slow and controlled.

inhale ▶ exhale inhale ‖ ▶ ‖

ball cable fly

pectorals and deltoids

Like the Cable crossover (see pages 80–81) this exercise works the pectoral muscles in your chest and the anterior deltoids at the front of your shoulders. You will need a ball for this exercise.

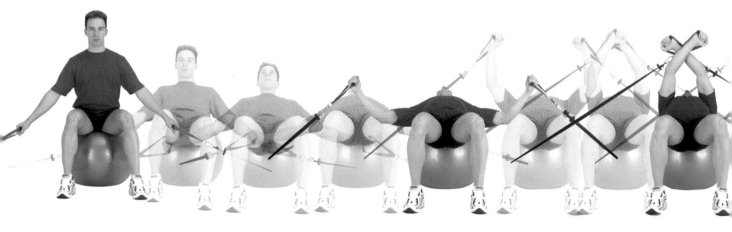

● This exercise uses the lower cable pulley. Position yourself and the ball in the center of the cable columns. To set up, begin by sitting on the ball, holding it at the sides. Walk your feet forward, rolling the ball beneath your lower back.

● Continue to roll the ball until you are lying down face upward with your upper back, shoulders and head resting on the ball. Your feet should be flat against the floor and your knees bent at a 90 degree angle.

● Your arms should be extended but soft at the elbows, hands gripping the cable handles with your palms facing toward the ceiling.

● Take your hands up toward the ceiling. Be careful not to lift your back as you perform this move. The movement should be isolated in the arms and shoulders.

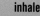 **begin to inhale** ▶ **inhale** ▶ **begin to exhale** ▶

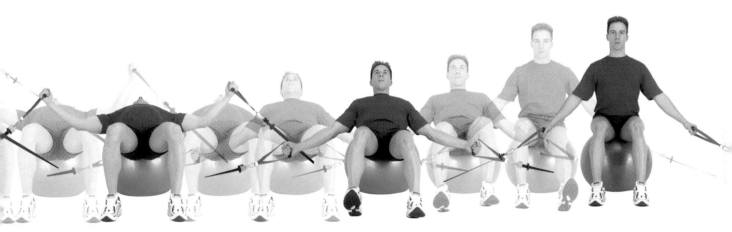

● As you reach full flexion your hands cross over each other. Cross your wrists over each other and do not strain any further.

● Hold the position for a moment, then start to take your arms back down again toward the floor. Keep your knees bent and your back resting on the ball.

● Keep the movement smooth and flowing as you return to the start position. Now repeat this arm exercise as many times as is comfortable.

● When you have finished, keep hold of the handles and gradually lean forward, pushing yourself up to a sitting position. Be careful not to strain your neck as you come up.

exhale ▶ **inhale** exhale ▶ **II**

reverse fly
rhomboids and deltoids

This exercise will test your rhomboids, posterior deltoids, and trapezius muscles in your shoulders and upper back. This exercise is the opposite of the Cable crossover (see pages 80–81) in that the movement is outward and upward.

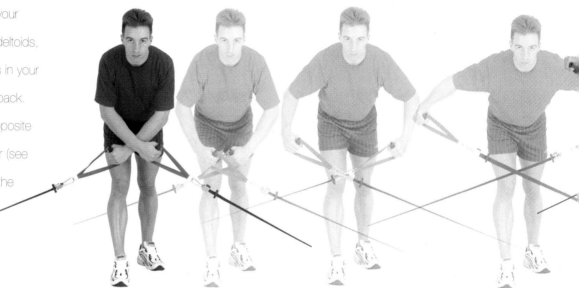

● This exercise uses the lower cable pulley. To set up, stand in the middle of the two cable columns, in line with the columns. Step forward with your right leg and lean forward to support your body weight.

● Now grip the two cable handles from the opposite sides. Begin the exercise by slowly pulling outward and upward. Make sure that you keep your arms roughly aligned throughout the movement.

● Continue to pull until your chest is fully expanded. Lean forward to gain a full contraction. Be careful not to hunch your shoulders as you bring your arms up toward the ceiling.

❚❚ inhale ▶ begin to exhale ▶ exhale ▶

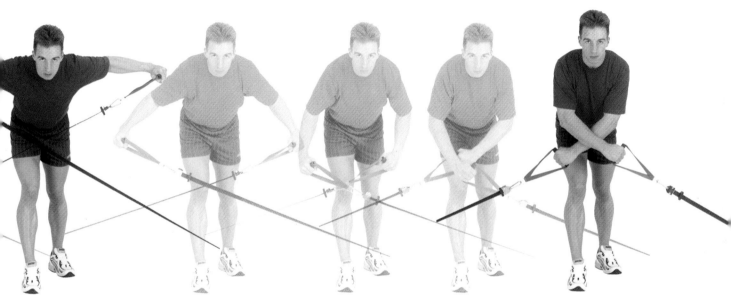

● Bring your arms up so that they are at a 90 degree angle to your body. Remember to keep your abdominal muscles tight to provide support for your lower back.

● Now release the cables and lower your arms back down again toward the floor. Keep your torso and legs stable and supportive.

● Return your arms back to the start position, crossing them over in front of your body. Keep your head facing forward and don't allow the neck to drop.

● Repeat the exercise as many times as necessary. Remember to keep the movement slow, controlled, and flowing.

inhale ▶ exhale inhale ‖ ▶ ‖

front pushdown

latissimus dorsi and triceps

This exercise works the triceps and latissimus dorsi muscles in the upper back. You will need a cross bar attachment to perform this exercise.

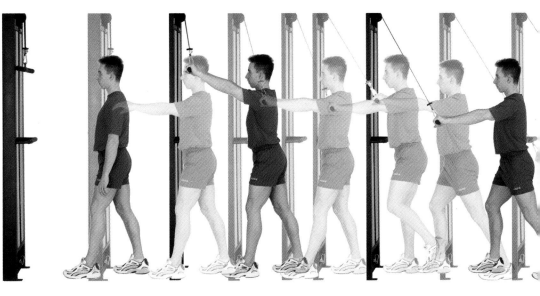

● Stand with your left leg 12 inches (30 centimeters) in front of one of the columns, and your right leg about 6 inches (15 centimeters) behind.

● Begin the pushdown with arms outstretched, making a 90 degree angle to the body. Depress the handles while keeping your arms straight. Push your chest out and your sternum upward as you perform the movement.

● Continue the downward movement, aiming your hands toward your body. Keep your shoulders back and don't become hunched. You will feel pressure around your chest, triceps, and shoulders.

| inhale | ▶ | start to exhale | ▶ | exhale | ▶ |

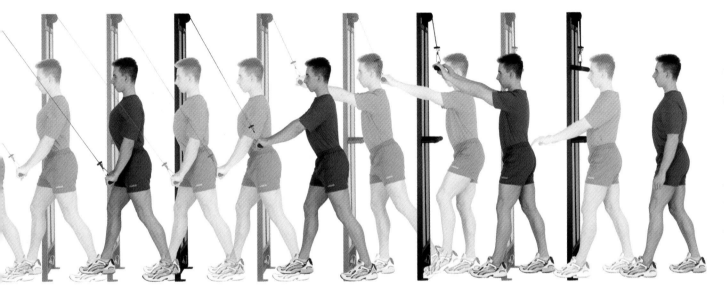

● Before you push the handles down, slowly move your left leg back so that it is stretched out behind you. Keep both knees soft and your heels on the floor as you perform this movement.

● Now slowly release the tension and raise the bar back up to the start position. Keep your abdominal muscles tensed throughout to ensure core stability.

● Repeat a number of pushdowns until you are tired. Be careful not to strain your arms and shoulders.

● If you want to increase the resistance for this exercise, step further back from the upright.

exhale   ▶   inhale   ❚❚   ▶   ■

low row rhomboids and biceps

This exercise will work your biceps and the muscles of your
upper back—the latissimus dorsi and rhomboids.

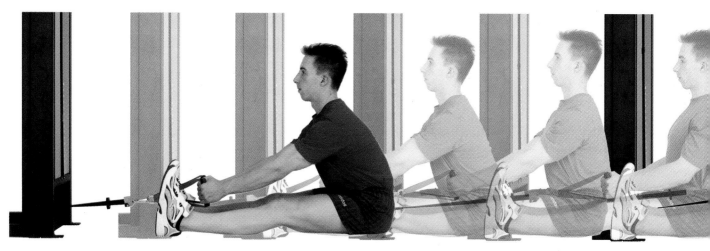

● This exercise uses the lower cable pulley. To set up, sit in front facing the cable column. Grip the cable handles with both hands. Sit at a distance so that you will have to lean forward to grip the handles.

● Rest your feet against a bar or footrest to bear the strain and provide stability for the movement. Your legs should be straight, but not locked at the knees.

● To begin the exercise, exhale and pull the cable handles back slowly to bear the tension. With elbows soft, pull from the arms. Keep your back, neck and head straight throughout the movement, and extend from the hips.

● Continue to pull until the handles rest against your upper abdomen. Pull with your upper back (rhomboids)— do not pull from the hands, as you will only be working the biceps.

■   **inhale** ▶ **exhale** ▶ **inhale** ▶

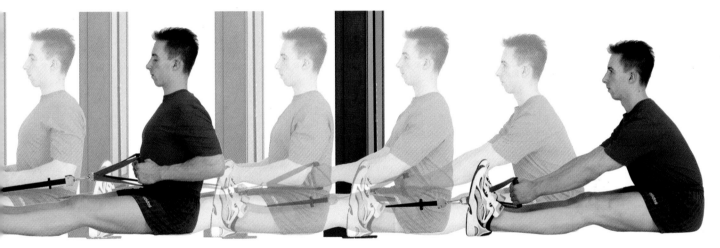

● Only pull yourself to an upright position—do not extend beyond 90 degrees as this could strain your lower back. Take your shoulders back. You will feel a contraction in your sides and upper back.

● Now inhale and release the tension in the cable, slowly letting it move back to the start position. Keep your back straight throughout, making sure that you bend from the hips.

● Keep your forearms level and parallel to the floor throughout the movement and make sure you keep your legs flat on the floor. As you pull the handles toward you, make sure that your shoulders are relaxed and not hunched.

● Repeat the movement as many times as is comfortable, taking care not to strain your back or shoulders in any way.

exhale   ▶   **inhale**   **exhale**   ‖   ▶   ‖

deltoid raise *and trapezius*

This is a harder version of the lateral raises with dumbbells (pages 32–33).

It will work your shoulder muscles (medial deltoids) and the trapezius muscle in the upper back and neck.

● Note that the cable deltoid raise is much harder than the dumbbell raise because the resistance is constant throughout. In the dumbbell raise, the greatest resistance is in the final part of the movement.

● This exercise uses the lower cable pulley. To set up, stand in the middle of the cable columns. Space your feet widely apart, with your left foot slightly forward to protect your back and to focus the movement in the shoulders.

● Begin with your hands relaxed and holding the handles in a cross over position. Gradually take up the tension and bring your hands apart and away from the body.

● Move your arms up toward the ceiling, keeping your arms facing forward and your elbows bent. Keep your body stable and your back straight throughout the movement. Raise your arms so that they are level with your shoulders.

| **inhale** ▶ | **exhale** ▶ | **inhale** ▶ |

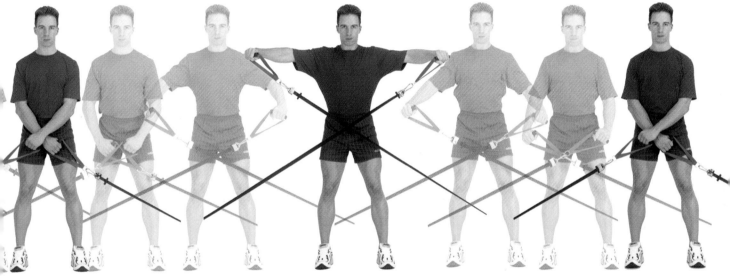

● Keep your elbows slightly higher than your hands throughout the movement (this ensures that you are exercising your shoulder muscles).

● Then inhale and slowly return your arms back toward the floor again. When repeating the exercise do not let the cable go slack, but continue the raises without crossing your hands.

● To complete an advanced variation, extend your arms fully, while keeping your elbows soft, so that they are at full contraction—90 degrees to the body. Remember not to hunch your shoulders as you raise your arms up.

● Repeat either exercise as many times as necessary, taking care not to strain your back or shoulder muscles.

exhale   ▶ inhale   exhale   ‖   ▶   ‖

ball shoulder press *deltoids and torso*

This is an advanced exercise that works your deltoids. The ball provides extra resistance by forcing the body to maintain balance throughout the movement.

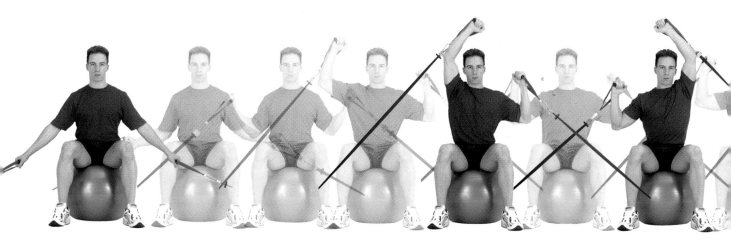

● This exercise uses the lower cable pulley. To set up, sit on the ball in the middle of the cable column with your feet flat on the ground and knees firm.

● Lift both hands up so that they are roughly in line with your head. Your arms will be bent at the elbows at a 45 degree angle and your palms will face inward toward your body.

● Now begin the exercise by pushing your right hand upward and inward toward the top of your head. You will need to rotate your palm outward as you perform this move.

● Raise your arm so that it is over your head. Then bring the arm back down again and repeat this movement with your left arm.

| inhale | ▶ | start to exhale | ▶ | exhale | ▶ |

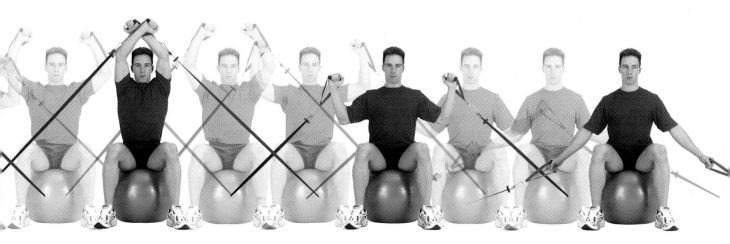

● Alternatively, you can raise both arms upward and inward toward each other. Keep your elbows aligned and level throughout the raise. Keep your upper body stable and firm throughout and do not arch your back as you push.

● Extend until your arms cross over in the center. You will feel pressure on your shoulders. Hold the pose briefly. Remember not to hunch your shoulders or lean back.

● Now inhale and slowly lower your hands back to the start position, with palms facing inward toward the body. Keep your head facing forward and be careful not to tense your neck.

● Repeat the exercise either one arm at a time or both together. To perform a more difficult variation, extend your arms fully as you reach up.

inhale ▶ exhale inhale ‖ ▶ ‖

cable biceps curl

This is a primary exercise for working the biceps and performs the same function as the Standing biceps curl on pages 38–39. However, using the cable for this workout provides constant resistance so this routine is a more advanced version. The latissimus dorsi and triceps are also engaged as they act as stabilizing muscles.

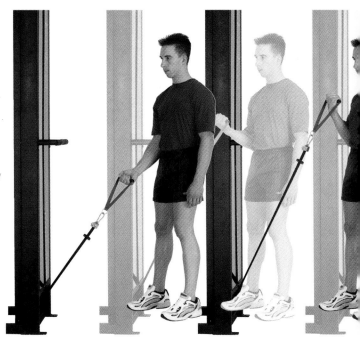

● Hold the handle in your right hand with palm facing upward and your lower arm extended to a soft position, taking the tension in the cable. To begin the exercise, flex your elbow to raise your hand up toward your shoulder.

● Keep your upper body stable and your knees soft. Remember not to lean back to assist in the lift. Keep your latissimus dorsi and triceps tight throughout to concentrate the tension on the biceps.

▶ **inhale**   **start to exhale**   ▶   **exhale**   ▶

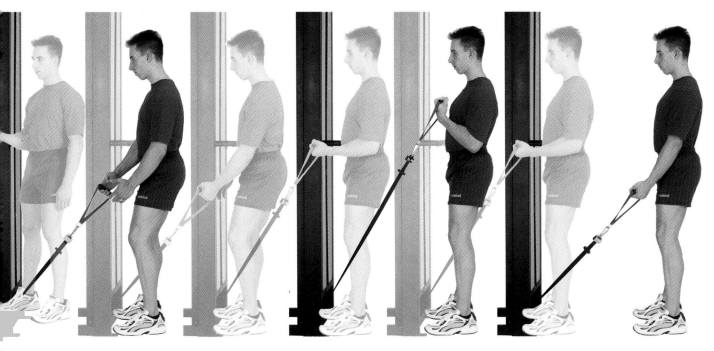

● Continue the movement until your palm is facing inward and the bicep is fully flexed and you cannot move it any further.

● Now extend your arm and lower the handle to the start position. Repeat the exercise without letting the tension go from the cable pulley. Do as many repetitions as is required. Be careful not to strain your arms or back.

● Then change hands and begin the bicep curl with your left arm. Remember to keep your knees soft and your legs hip's width apart.

● Repeat the exercise the same number of times with your left arm and then rest.

start to inhale ▶ inhale ‖ exhale ‖ ▶ ‖

cable curl with ball

This exercise will work and strengthen your biceps. It is essential that you set up this exercise correctly. You need to place the ball at a distance from the cable column so that when you come to raise the cable handle the strap is almost at a 45 degree angle from the floor.

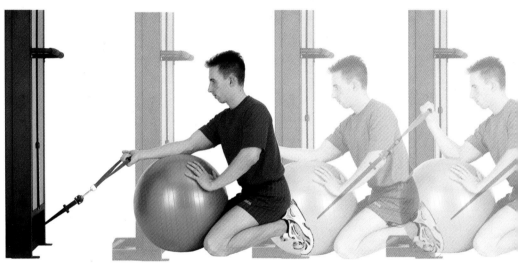

● Kneel, facing the upright. Have your knees on the ground and curl your toes under. Tuck your knees in tightly to the ball and rest your right arm on the top of the ball. Hold the cable handle with palm facing upward.

● Your elbow should be centrally positioned on top of the ball. The ball provides extra resistance and helps to isolate the bicep for a good workout. Place your resting hand on the side of the ball for additional balance.

● Flexing at the elbow, raise your right arm to take the tension. To begin the exercise, exhale and flex your arm, bringing it slowly up toward your body.

| start to inhale | ▶ | inhale | ▶ | start to exhale | ▶ |

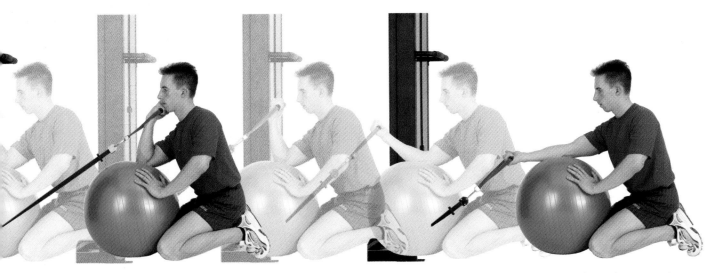

● Continue to raise the handle until your biceps are fully flexed. Keep your body firm and your knees tucked into the ball for stability.

● Inhale and begin to lower your arm back to the start position. Keep your body still and don't tense the neck.

● Lower your arm slowly and concentrate on keeping your elbow steady. Keep your shoulders relaxed. Inhale as you bring the arm down.

● Repeat this exercise as many times as is required. Then change arms and begin the routine flexing the elbow and working the muscles in your left arm.

exhale ▶ exhale inhale ‖ ▶ ‖

tricep rope pushdown

This exercise works your triceps. The latissimus dorsi are also engaged as they act as stabilizing muscles during the workout.

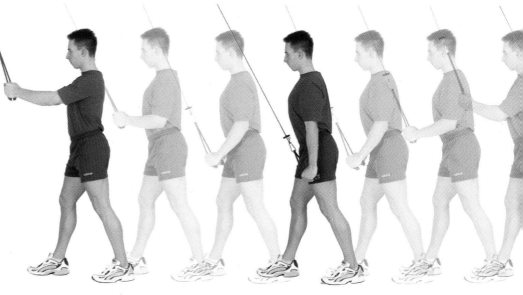

● To set up, stand approximately 12 inches (30 centimeters) in front of one of the cable columns, with your right foot in front of your left one and both feet positioned firmly. Your legs should be firm, but slightly soft at the knees.

● Using both arms, pull the rope attachment downward until your arms are roughly 90 degrees to the body, or parallel to the floor. This is the start position.

● To begin the exercise, push downward, bending at the elbows. You will need to contract your latissimus dorsi to keep your upper body stable. Don't lean forward to use your body to push down the rope—the movement is in the arms.

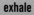 inhale ▶ exhale ▶ inhale ▶

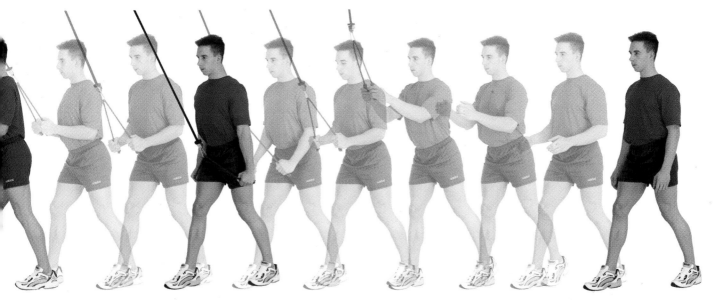

● Continue the move downward, gradually parting your hands as your arms extend. Your forearms will twist slightly on the downward movement. Complete the extension with elbows locked and arms fully extended.

● Now raise your hands back up to the start position, 90 degrees from the body. Be careful not to arch the back as you raise your hands up again.

● Lower your arms back down to your sides again and then up toward the ceiling to complete another repetition. Keep the movement slow and controlled.

● When you have finished this exercise, let go of the rope attachment and relax your arms by your sides.

exhale   ▶ **inhale**   **exhale**   ❚❚   ▶   ■

triceps cable kickback

This exercise works the triceps in just the same way as the Triceps kickback (see pages 38–39), although it is a slightly harder workout since the pressure on the muscles is maintained by the cable's tension right from the beginning.

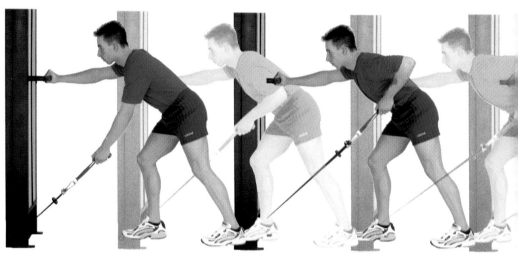

● To set up for the triceps kickback, face toward the column and step your left foot backward to get into a low position. Lean forward, extend your right arm and hold on to the bar with your hand for stability and to bear your body weight.

● Make sure you keep both knees soft during this exercise and keep your feet flat on the floor. The movement should be isolated in the arm and your body should remain still.

● Holding the cable, extend your left arm until it is parallel to the floor, keeping your upper arm rigid. Your extended upper arm must remain stable at all times.

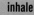 **start to inhale** ▶ **inhale** ▶ **start to exhale** ▶

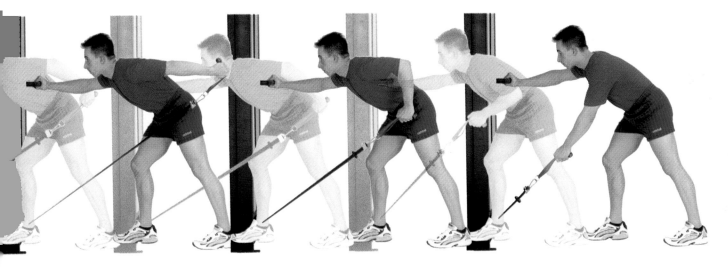

● Keep your back straight throughout the exercise. Remember not to twist or rotate your body when extending your arm.

● Now inhale and flex your forearm to return to the start position, allowing the cable tension to bring your arm back toward the column.

● Repeat the movement a number of times without straining your arm. Make sure you don't hunch your shoulders at any point during this exercise and that your neck is relaxed.

● Now do the triceps extension using the right arm and stabilizing your body weight with your extended left arm.

exhale ▶ **inhale** **exhale** ‖ ▶ ‖

triceps extension with ball

This exercise works the triceps by gaining extra leverage from the ball. The use of the ball also helps to isolate the movement in your upper arms to increase flexibility and strength.

● This exercise can use the middle or the upper cable pulley. To set up, kneel behind the ball, facing away from the cable column. Tuck your knees under the ball for stability.

● Using your right hand, grip the handle from the cable behind you. Make sure you are far enough away from the column to feel tension in the cable.

● Center your elbows on the top of the ball, using the ball for extra leverage. To start the exercise, exhale and begin to extend your right arm forward toward the floor.

● Continue the downward extension so that your forearm slowly rotates and your palm points downward. Remember to keep your body firm and stable throughout to concentrate the tension on the triceps.

| inhale | ▶ | start to exhale | ▶ | exhale | ▶ |

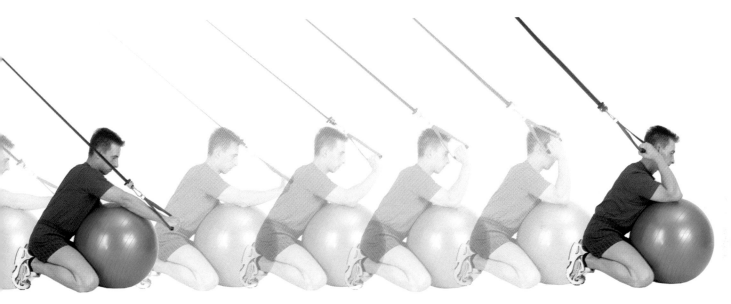

● Complete the extension with your palm pointed forward and your arm pushing so that it is fully extended. Keep your back straight and do not allow your neck to become tense.

● Now slowly return your right arm to the start position. Make sure that your elbow remains still and the movement is isolated in the arm.

● As you bring the arm back up again, twist your fist slowly around toward your body so that your palm is facing inward again. Repeat the exercise a number of times taking care not to strain your arm.

● Now, using your left arm, repeat the exercise. Make sure you do the same number of repetitions as you practiced with your right arm.

exhale ▶ inhale exhale ❚❚ ▶ ❚❚

cable crunch with ball

This exercise will work your rectus abdominis muscles, which when developed appear as a series of ripples, or "six pack," on the surface of the stomach. You will need good torso strength to perform this exercise.

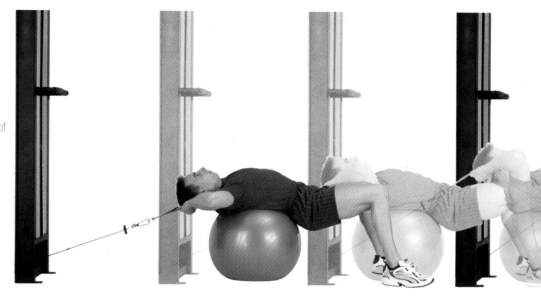

● Get into position so that your upper back is resting on the ball with your knees bent at 90 degrees and your feet flat on the floor. Your knees will need to remain firm throughout the exercise to provide stability.

● Gripping the cable handle tightly with both hands, hold it behind the back of your head. You should be at a distance from the cable upright so that as soon as you lift your body the cable will become tense.

● To begin the exercise, exhale and flex your body from the abdomen. Pull yourself forward in a smooth, rolling movement toward your legs—not upward toward the ceiling.

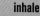

start to inhale ▶ inhale ▶ begin to exhale ▶

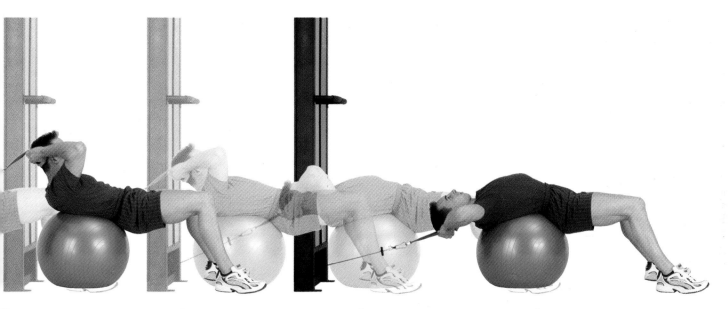

● Continue the flexion until your abdominals are compressed. The stabilizing muscles are essential in this movement, as you must maintain balance and stability and concentrate all the pressure on the abdominals.

● Now lower yourself slowly back down to the start position in a smooth, rolling movement. Keep your knees bent to help with your balance and don't let your neck drop.

● Repeat the exercise as many times as is comfortable without straining your lower back or abdomen.

● This is a safe abdominal exercise because the ball supports and protects your lower back while allowing you to concentrate on your abdominal muscles.

exhale   ▶   inhale   ❚❚   ▶   ❚❚

back extensions with ball

A counterpoise to the Cable crunch exercise (see pages 104–105), this is an advanced exercise
that will work your lower back while providing safe support with the ball.

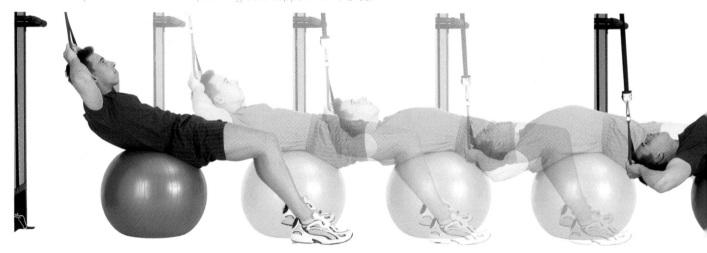

● This exercise uses the upper cable pulley. To set up, face away from the cable column. Lean back on the ball and roll the ball beneath your body pushing against the soles of your feet.

● Get into position so that your upper back is resting on the ball with your knees bent at 90 degrees and your feet flat on the floor and splayed apart for balance. Your knees will need to remain firm to provide stability.

● Gripping the cable handle tightly with both hands, hold it against the top of your head. You should be at a distance from the cable upright so that as soon as you pull on the cable you will feel resistance.

● To begin the exercise, slowly extend your body toward the floor, keeping your hands on your head. All the resistance will be from above, so you will need to pull downward.

▶ **inhale** ▶ **start to exhale** ▶

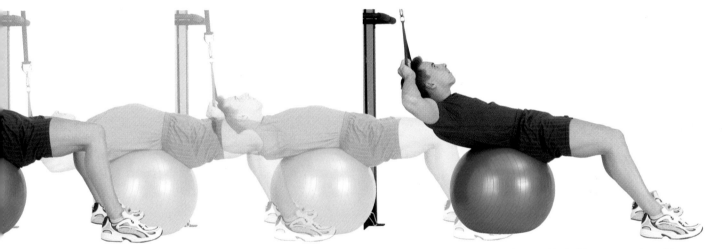

● Continue to pull downward as far as possible. Keep your knees firm for stability and balance. Make sure that you don't drop your neck.

● Now begin to raise your body back up to the start position. Be careful not to raise it too high—just so that your shoulders are lifted from the ball. Remember to keep your elbows still and not bent in toward your body.

● Repeat the extension a number of times without straining your arms or back in any way, then relax.

● The ball is an extremely useful element in this exercise as it provides a pivot point that supports the back, which also improves safety and reduces the risk of injury.

exhale ▶ inhale exhale ▶ **11**

kneeling crunch

This routine consists of two exercises that will give your torso a good workout—the kneeling forward crunch flattens, tones, and strengthens the abdominal muscles, while the side crunch works the external and internal obliques.

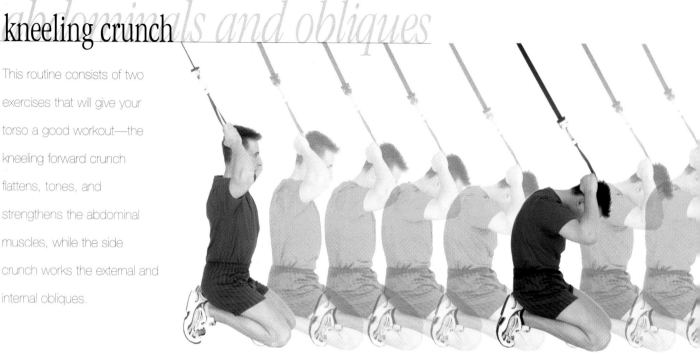

● Kneel in front of the cable column, facing away from the weights. Hold the cable handle behind the back of your head, gripping tightly with your fingers. Your hands should form a "hook" to which you can then attach the cable pulley.

● To perform the forward crunch, bend downward, slowly rolling your body in a downward motion. It is important that you bend downward to work the abdomen, as if you bend forward, you will be placing pressure on your lower back.

● Keep bending while looking down toward the floor. Now inhale and return to the start position. Repeat the movement without straining your abdomen.

| inhale | ▶ | exhale | ▶ | inhale | ▶ |

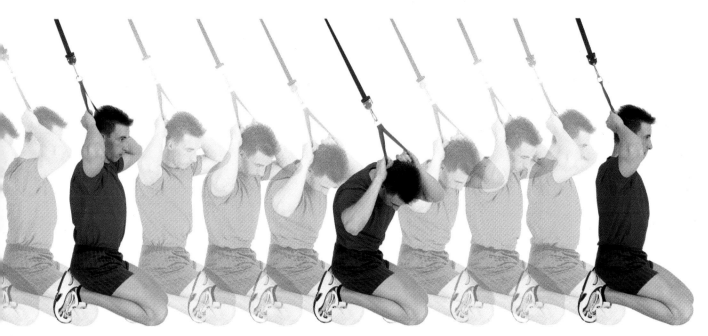

● To perform the side crunch, use the same set up position, kneeling on your haunches and balancing on your toes. Hold the cable handle behind the back of your head, gripping tightly with your fingers.

● Now bend downward, but twisting your body to the right side in a slow rolling motion. Again, keep bending downward looking toward the floor.

● Bend as far as you can, then come up to the start position. Repeat the side bend as many times as possible without straining.

● Return to the start position and then repeat the side crunch to your left side. Perform the same number of repetitions as you practiced with your right side.

exhale ▶ inhale exhale ‖ ▶ ‖

ball twist

transversus abdominis

This exercise works the transversus abdominis muscle, beneath the diaphragm in the upper

abdomen. Be careful not to strain your abdomen when performing this routine.

● This exercise uses the lower cable pulley. To set up, sit on the center of the ball facing forward with the cable column to your right. Sitting on the ball will force the upper body muscles to keep the torso tensed and upright.

● Position your feet flat on the floor 18 inches (45 centimeters) apart. Take your left arm across the body and take hold of the handles with both hands.

● To begin the exercise, pull the cable across the body with arms fully extended and soft at the elbows. Your arms and shoulders act as a lever for your abdominal muscles.

● The movement will make an arc from the lower right to the upper left. Continue the movement until your hands are extended and roughly at head height on your left-hand side.

inhale ▶ **start to exhale** ▶ **exhale** ▶

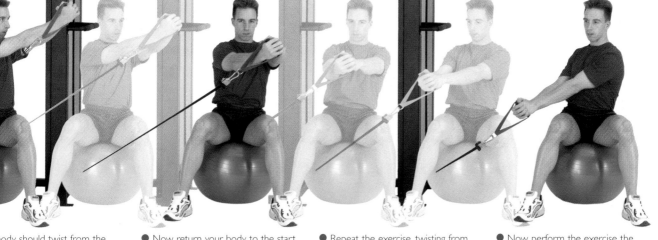

● Your body should twist from the waist. You are performing the exercise incorrectly if you only move your arms.

● Now return your body to the start position, letting the cable tension pull you to the bottom right. Remember to keep your elbows and shoulders stiff and soft throughout the movement.

● Repeat the exercise, twisting from the waist. You should feel a tightness around your upper abdomen and sides. Repeat a number of times without over-working your arms or shoulders.

● Now perform the exercise the same amount of times on the other side, taking care not to strain your abdomen.

exhale ▶ inhale ‖ exhale ▶ ‖

side bends *quadratus lumborum*

This routine tones and strengthens the oblique muscles (located at the sides of your waist) through a sideways flexion. It also works the quadratus lumborum muscle.

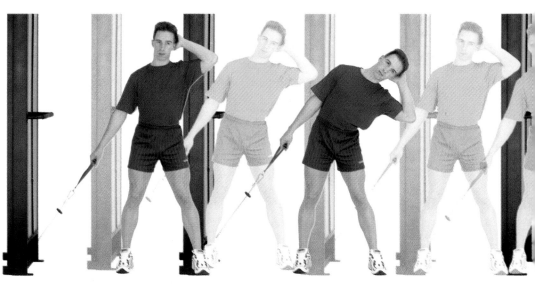

● Stand at a distance where you feel immediate tension from the cable. The arm holding the cable should be relaxed and not taking the pressure. Place your resting hand on the back of your head.

● To begin the exercise, extend your upper body away from the cable, bending from the waist. The pressure should be on the sides of your torso—do not pull the cable with your hands, but merely use your arm as a lever.

● Extend your body as far as you can away from the machine, then slowly bend back toward the machine. As you return you will feel a contraction on your left side that is caused by the resistance.

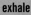 **inhale** ▶ **exhale** ▶ **inhale** ▶

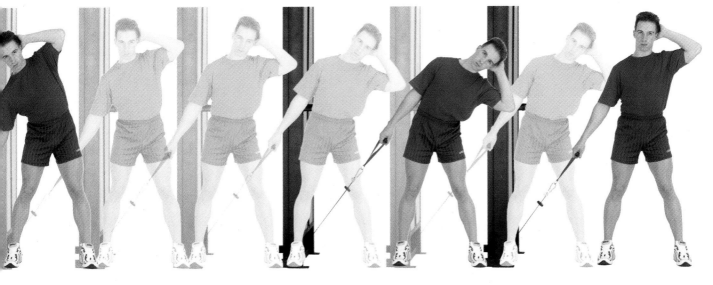

● Remember to keep your hips square at all times and do not twist your body.

● Continue the sideways movement from side to side without straining. You will also feel a compression on the right side when returning your body to the right.

● Do as many repetitions as is required. Keep your head facing forward and your lower body still. Concentrate on isolating the movement in your waist.

● If performed slowly and carefully, this exercise is a safe and effective way to tone and strengthen the obliques.

exhale ▶ inhale ‖ ▶ ‖

rotator cuff

This works the shoulders' rotator cuffs—the inner shoulder muscles. The shoulder joints are one of the weakest in the body because of their shallow sockets, so it is important to strengthen them.

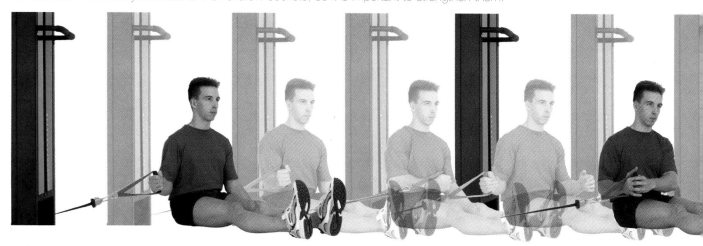

● This exercise can use both the lower and middle pulley. Make sure you are sitting far enough away from the pulley so you feel resistance when gripping the cable handle.

● Keep your upper body rigid and flex your latissimus dorsi and triceps to provide stability for this exercise. Align the cable handle with your elbow, slightly behind your hand.

● Slowly pull your right arm into the body. Make sure you pivot from the elbow and keep your upper arm steady and close to your side. Rotate as far as your can, concentrating all the effort in your shoulder.

● Return the cable to the start position and change hands to exercise the other shoulder.

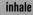

inhale　　　　　　　　**exhale**　　▶　　**inhale**　　▶　　**begin to exhale**　　▶

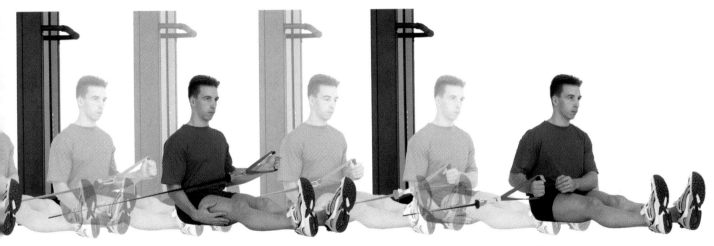

● Remember to keep your back straight as you pull the cable handle away from your body. Do not hunch your shoulders as you exercise them.

● Keep your upper arm steady and close to your side as you concentrate all the effort in your left shoulder. Be careful not to tense the neck.

● Return the pulley back to its start position and change hands again. Make sure you align the cable handle with your elbow again before starting the pull.

● If you want less resistance, you can change the cable from the lower pulley to the middle one.

exhale　　　　**exhale**　▶　**begin to inhale**　▶　**inhale**

chin ups

and latissimus dorsi

This is a very traditional exercise for working and strengthening the biceps and latissimus dorsi muscles. There are two potential positions for chin ups, a narrow grip and wide grip. The narrow position gives more peak to the biceps, while the wider grip works and expands the latissimus dorsi muscles.

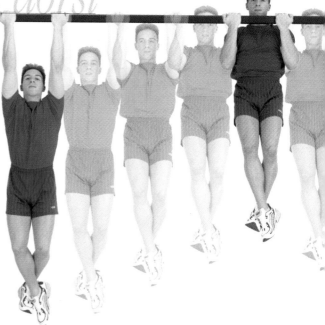

● To take up the narrow grip position for this exercise, reach up to hold the bar with your palms facing inward and your arms about shoulder width apart.

● Cross your ankles to stop them swinging freely and to increase stability. Throughout the movement, keep your back and legs as rigid as possible to aid a smooth rise and fall.

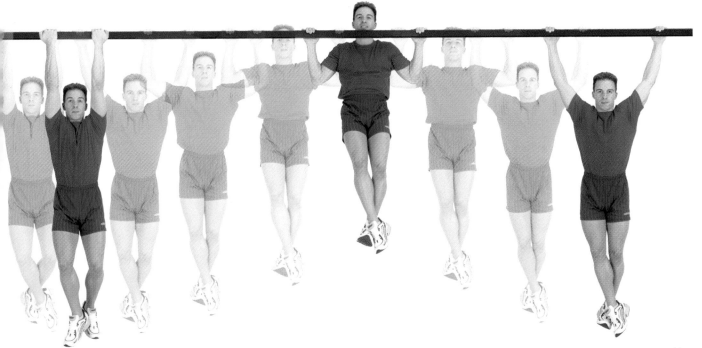

● Now pull yourself up to the bar as far as you can, dipping your chin over the bar, before slowly lowering yourself to the start position. Repeat as many times as possible.

● For the wide position, extend your arms in a "V" shape, palms facing forward, and grip the bar. Your hands should be roughly the same width apart as your elbows when extended laterally.

● Again, cross your ankles to stop them swinging freely and to increase stability. Now pull yourself up to the bar as far as you can, dipping your chin over the bar if possible.

● Lower yourself to the start position again. You will feel a contraction in the latissimus dorsi muscles in your back. Repeat the movement as many times as possible without straining.

exhale   ▶   inhale   exhale   ▶   ‖

reverse upright row

trapezius and deltoids

This exercise works the trapezius muscle in the upper back and neck, and the posterior and medial deltoid muscles in the shoulders.

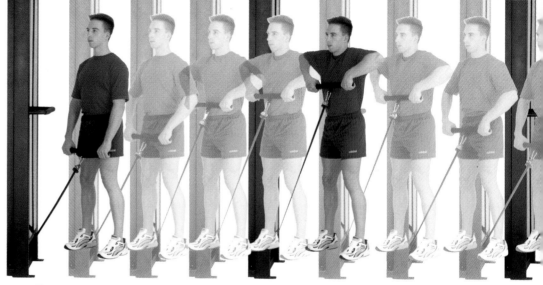

● To set up, stand in front of the cable column, with your feet splayed roughly 18 inches (45 centimeters) apart and positioned firmly. Your legs should be firm, but slightly soft at the knees.

● Stand far enough away from the cable column to take up the tension. Now, using both arms, lift up the bar, keeping your hands, elbows and forearms parallel to the body.

● Continue the movement until your shoulders and upper arms are about 90 degrees to the body. Throughout the movement your elbows should rotate upward and your hands should rotate downward.

inhale ▶ **start to exhale** ▶ **exhale** ▶

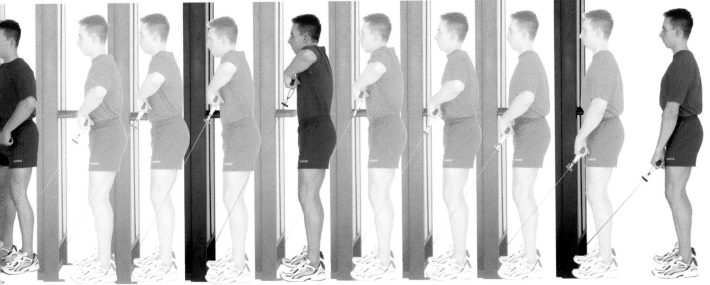

● Hold the position briefly, but do not let your hands go higher than your elbows, as this can strain the wrists. Do not allow your neck to become tense as you raise your arms.

● Now lower the bar back down to the start position, and repeat the exercise as many times as required.

● Keep your back straight as you perform this exercise and try not to hunch your shoulders as you raise your arms.

● When you have finished this exercise place the bar attachment gently on the floor and relax.

inhale ▶ exhale inhale ‖ ▶ ‖

reverse cable curl

This exercise will work the hip flexors and abdominal muscles, and

increase the strength in these areas.

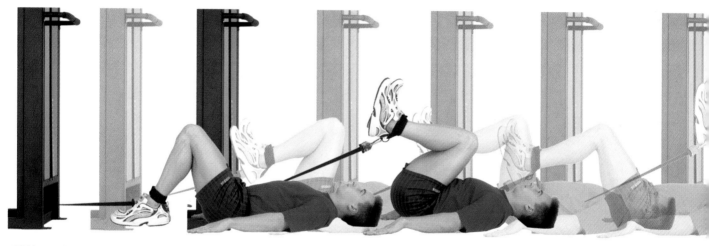

● This exercise uses the lower cable pulley. First, tie your ankles together with an ankle cable so that your feet are close but not uncomfortable.

● Lie flat on the floor, facing toward the cable upright, with your arms flat against the floor for support and balance. Lie at a distance that allows you to take up the cable tension as soon as you raise your legs.

● To begin the exercise, tilt your hips toward your chest and then bring your knees toward your chest too. Keep your feet and legs suspended throughout the movement.

● Continue to flex at the hips and contract into your chest as far as is comfortable. Keep the movement slow and controlled without straining your ankles.

inhale ▶ start to exhale ▶ exhale ▶

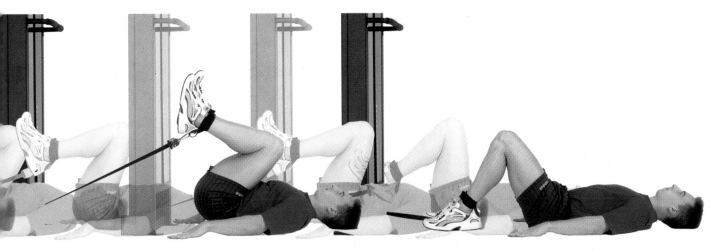

● Now bring your lower legs back out from the body toward the floor, keeping your knees bent. Remember to keep your back flat against the floor throughout the exercise. If arching occurs, check that it is pain free.

● Bring your knees back in toward your chest again. Keep your arms flat on the floor to help you balance.

● Make sure your head remains on the floor as you move your knees and that your back does not strain at any time.

● Repeat the contractions as many times as is comfortable and then rest with your knees bent and your feet flat on the floor.

inhale ▶ exhale inhale ❚❚ ▶ ■

treadmill *muscles*

Running on a treadmill is a great cardiovascular workout, and exercises almost all of the leg muscles as well as keeping the back and abdominal muscles tight. It is also a good way to ensure minimal impact damage.

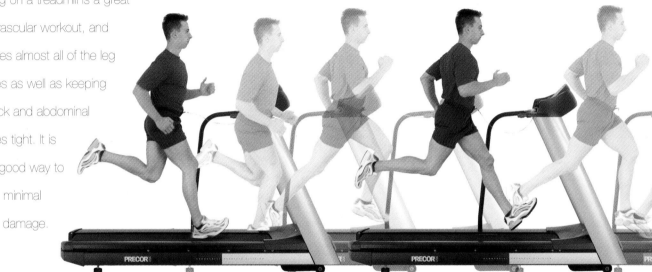

● Treadmills are cushioned, flat, safe, all-weather alternatives to outdoor running. Regular runners should wear proper running shoes with cushioned soles that are designed to stand up to the stresses of running.

● Before beginning a run, stretch your legs and loosen your joints and muscles (see page 14).

● Stand on the treadmill. Attach the safety cord to the front of your shorts or running pants. This will stop you losing balance and will help you maintain a correct position on the machine without rolling off.

● Switch the machine on and begin exercising at a walking pace. Continue walking for a few minutes until you have warmed up and your muscles feel looser.

■   inhale   ▶   exhale   ▶   inhale   ▶

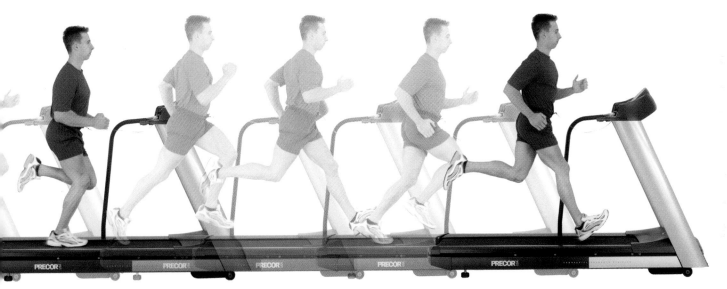

● Speed up the pace and lengthen your strides to a fast walk. From the longer strides, gradually pick up the pace and begin to run. Build up to the running pace gradually to allow your muscles to adjust to the movement.

● You can run at many different paces, depending on whether you want to concentrate on increasing your endurance or improving your speed. Some runners measure their progress with a heart rate monitor.

● Speedwork—fast repetitions interspersed with slower periods—can improve strength and speed, and increase running efficiency. Longer, slower runs will increase endurance, build muscles, and burn calories.

● Do not push yourself too hard when running—if you feel any strain or discomfort, abort the session immediately. Running on injured muscles can do more damage and increase the time it takes to recover.

exhale ▶ inhale exhale ▶ ‖

efx machine

You can exercise most of the main muscle groups with an EFX (Elliptical Fitness Crosstraining) machine, making it ideal for a whole body workout.

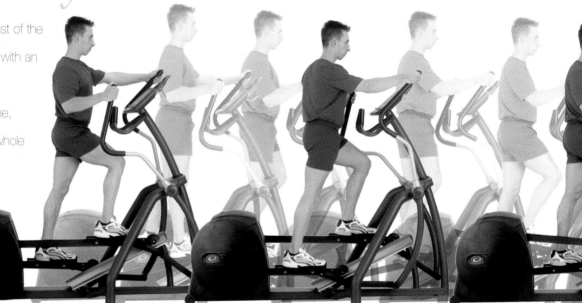

● An EFX machine is a good way of warming up in preparation for other kinds of exercise. The elliptical motion works the whole body by maintaining resistance through the handlebars and steps on both the arms and legs.

● There are two main techniques for using an EFX machine, one easy and one more difficult. You can choose a technique according to your needs.

● To practice the difficult technique, take up a squatting pose, keeping your back as upright as possible. Push with your legs and arms. This pose puts greater stress on your legs and arms, as all the weight is on these limbs.

● This advanced position involves much greater body tension and places pressure on the quadriceps and hips to hold the body in position when you are pushing.

inhale ▶ exhale ▶ inhale ▶

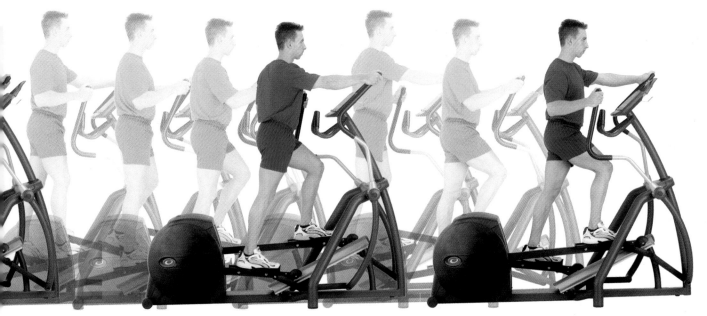

● To practice the simpler technique, stand upright on the machine and push downward with your legs. This will create a rising and falling motion that is easier on the body, as you can move in rhythm with the machine.

● On many machines, you can practice a forward or reverse stride, as well as adjust the handlebars to vary the workout and emphasize different muscle groups.

● The steps and handlebars also allow you to concentrate your workout on either the leg or arm muscles. To work the legs, rest your hands on the hand grip. To work the arms, focus on pushing and pulling the handles.

● Regular practice with an EFX machine is also an excellent way to become fitter while overcoming injuries, since the motion does not place excessive stress on any particular joints or muscles.

exhale   ▶   **inhale**   **exhale**   ▶   **II**

index

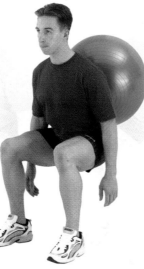